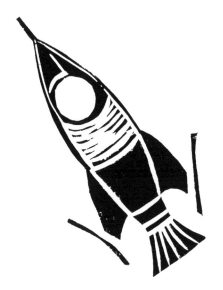

WE BEAT LEUKAEMIA

MELODY BERTHOUD

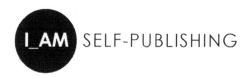

SELF-PUBLISHING

🐦 @iamselfpub
www.iamselfpublishing.com

For Andrew and Clara

I love you a bushel and a peck

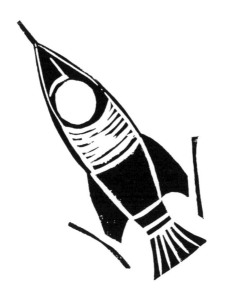

WE BEAT
LEUKAEMIA

"When you launch in a rocket, you're not really flying that rocket. You're just sort of hanging on."

Michael P. Anderson – NASA astronaut

Contents

Chapter 1

Diagnosis

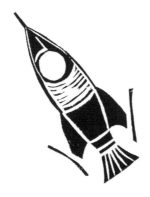

Ev'ry parent's thought

Not my son, my world, my child

I wish it were me.

Andrew was born in May 2009 in time for afternoon tea. It was a gorgeous summer's day and the multi coloured tulips in our garden were in full bloom. My husband, Joseph, raced home to collect Clara, aged two. She arrived shyly in the hospital room and was introduced to her baby brother. Two years before, when I was pregnant with Clara, I left my deputy head role to become a stay at home mum. I thoroughly enjoyed the life of coffee mornings, play dates in the garden, toddler groups and classes which punctuated our week.

In May 2012 the tulips were in bloom again. Andrew celebrated his third birthday and Clara had already turned five. It was the summer of the 2012 London Olympics and we had won three sets of tickets in the ballot for basketball, hockey and volleyball. We decided to staycate that summer, rather than go abroad, and enjoy the buzz and atmosphere in London. Joseph and I started to make plans about my return to work. We decided I could go back to work regularly for two days a week so I was delighted to be offered a part time job as a primary consultant for a multi academy trust in London, starting in September 2012.

On my first day back at work, with butterflies in my stomach and new shoes on my feet, I got the train to Peckham Rye and felt such a sense of excitement, liberation and freedom from my days at home as 'Mummy'. I walked past butcher shops with dead chickens hanging in their windows and revelled in the experience of going to different places, being with new colleagues and becoming Melody again.

One day when Clara was back at school, Andrew and I visited the London Transport Museum with friends. We had a lovely day out. We sat on the step in Covent Garden eating chocolate ice creams, the sun shining on our faces whilst watching an entertainer build up to his one and only unicycle trick. It was a lovely moment and I remember thinking how great life was. Everything was in balance.

Two weeks later however Andrew was not settled at pre-school. He was very tired, and on the days when I took him he refused to scoot, so I pulled him all the way. I would pre-empt his end of pre-school tiredness by picking him up with the pushchair and a sandwich, which he ate before falling asleep. At home he was listless and wanted to watch TV.

He started sweating at night and his pillow case was often wet in the morning – I thought nothing of it, as we were having a mild September. I turned his pillow over. He had a few nose bleeds in the night too, blood about the size of a fifty pence piece lying crimson on his pillowcase. Again I thought nothing of it; Joseph had suffered with nose bleeds as a child. I just stripped the pillow case and washed it.

A friend commented one afternoon at the school gate, when Andrew was fast asleep in the pushchair, that he was looking pale. Yes, I replied, he had been very tired recently and was probably sickening for something.

On Saturday 29th September 2012 Andrew woke up and was sick in the middle of the night. On Sunday 30th September we went to Coolings Nature Trail in Knockholt for some fresh air with my brother and his family. It was a lovely place with a short walk in the woods to look at some animals: a perfect outing for little legs. Andrew was still very tired. I hadn't taken the pushchair, as the ground was uneven, and I refused to carry Andrew, thinking he was being a lazy three-year-old. After all, everyone else was skipping and running about. He had to walk, I told him, otherwise he couldn't have a piece of cake in the café. My brother was a softer touch and picked him up. Andrew instantly fell asleep on his shoulder.

When Andrew developed a high temperature on Monday 1st October I wasn't surprised; he had been sickening for something. Here begins my Facebook diary of what happened next:

Monday, 1st October 2012
Cath – It was nice to see you and Laila at music class this morning – but antibac your phone, Andrew has a temp of 38.2!

Tuesday, 2nd October 2012
I am with Andrew in A&E at Queen Mary's Hospital, Sidcup.

Wednesday, 3rd October 2012
Andrew was diagnosed with leukaemia today. Curable. Such a brave boy.

Thanks to everyone for your kind messages, offers of help and support. We are moving to our new home at the Royal Marsden tomorrow where the chemotherapy will begin... I am finding it very hard to talk about, but it is much easier to converse in texts and emails.

Friday, 5th October 2012

Andrew and I are on the way to the Royal Marsden in Sutton and we are excited to have a ride in an ambulance.

The move to the Royal Marsden has been great. We have a private room, with facilities and professionals on every level. The Oak Centre for Children and Young people is an entire section of the hospital reserved for paediatric oncology. It was opened by Prince William a year ago, in September 2011. When we arrived Andrew was wheeled past a pool table, a juke box, a playroom, a school room. Everyone was welcoming and smiley. Once settled, we were given a tour of the facilities: there is a room with Miele washing machines and tumble driers; a parent's kitchen that provides tea, coffee, milk, bread, butter and jam every day for free, and I have paid the deposit to rent a small space in a huge fridge. The contrast to the facilities at the Queen Elizabeth, which is in administration, is stark.

Andrew is settled in an isolation room in case a spot on his tummy is chicken pox, (which would compromise everyone else here), but he is happy with the IPad, toys, DVDs, and magazines, and with Mummy and Daddy. We have our own bathroom and the green sofa doubles as a parent bed. Andrew is most excited about having a TV on the wall in his room.

The Doctor managed to get a cannula into his left arm after some numbing cream and several attempts. He has strapped it up really well with used plastic saline packets and bandages to protect it, so hopefully it will last. Nothing is being done until Tuesday when Andrew will have a bone marrow aspirate procedure, lumbar puncture and a portacath line fitted in his chest for the bloods and medicines.

Clara is coping well in the circumstances. We continue to be overwhelmed by the outpouring of love through texts, emails, cards and presents.

Saturday, 6th October 2012

There is no phone service in the leaded hospital, but there is Wi-Fi, which means we have internet and Facebook. I love reading what everyone else is up to. I have left a bag of library books needing to be returned on my windowsill if anyone is going past in the next few days. Andrew is asleep now but he is about to have a blood transfusion as his platelets are low. We have been told he could have an allergic reaction so I am hoping he doesn't. Otherwise everything is calm. The grandparents and Clara visited today.

Sunday, 7th October 2012

Joseph and I are at a Pub in Sutton. We are having a quick roast buffet lunch and much needed time to talk, thanks to both sets of grandparents. One set are in hospital with Andrew and the other at home with Clara. Joseph and I haven't spoken face to face to each other for more than five minutes since Andrew's diagnosis.

If we are both in hospital, we do not have time to talk as both the children demand our attention. We cannot talk in the evening as there is no phone signal in the room and we don't want to leave Andrew on his own. We have decided to try and Skype later tonight.

At home I used the book 'See Inside Your Body' by Usborne Books to explain about Andrew's poorly blood to Clara. There is a great page which explains about red blood cells, platelets and white bloods cells. It was very emotional explaining it all to Clara. I am not sure how much she understood.

Monday, 8th October 2012

I am back at the Royal Marsden with Andrew for my forty-eight-hour shift. Joseph has started writing down the key information from the doctors and nurses in a book, as the extreme tiredness makes it hard to remember what to say to each other when we swap shifts. The nurses are preparing Andrew for all the procedures tomorrow afternoon with a blood transfusion now. His saline fluid levels have been increased to flush out the high levels of phosphates found, so hourly trips to the loo are needed; otherwise all is 'normal'.

I found dropping Clara off to school upsetting this morning, especially when everyone was asking me about Andrew and how we are doing, so I am sorry if I ignored you whilst rushing home again. It is important for me to try and pretend everything is okay for the ten minutes needed to have Clara go in to school happily. Please feel free to email me or catch up on here about how we are doing and then hopefully I won't end up crying in the playground.

I stopped at Toys R Us on the way to the Royal Marsden to get a Batman for the Batcave here, the consultant told us not to spoil him, but it is very hard not to. You cannot ring or text me again but please keep in contact via Facebook.

Joseph and I managed to Skype each other tonight once both children were asleep. I talked softly so as not to wake Andrew, and plugged headphones in so I could hear Joseph. We found ourselves giggling at one point which felt so wrong but so right too.

Tuesday, 9th October 2012

It is nice to be home – it has been a tough day. Frequent loo trips and restless legs meant Andrew didn't sleep too well last night. He had a hearty breakfast but was Nil by Mouth after 8:15am, as we were due to go for his general anaesthetic at 2:30pm. He was going to be given the 'special sleep juice' through his cannula, but the cannula failed at about 1pm. The doctors removed it. They tried to reinsert another cannula for the hour or two before his op, but Andrew screamed, shouted and protested so much they couldn't. Thankfully they gave up and took him to the operation room anyway at 4pm. It was very distressing and I ended up in tears. Even one of the nurses left the room with tears in her eyes.

Andrew was amazing. In pre-op he drank the 'happy medicine,' which relaxed him. He then had the sleepy gas, through a mask, whilst playing a Toca Boca app on the registrar's IPhone. Joseph and I sat on a green chesterfield sofa outside the operation theatre, waiting. The operation was a success. Bone marrow aspirate, lumbar puncture and line are all done. Andrew was having such a lovely deep sleep he did not want to wake up. The great news is that the dermatologist said his skin lesion is not chicken pox or contagious and needs no further treatment other than moisturiser. As a result, we are now out of isolation, which means Andrew can leave the isolation room and have access to the playroom tomorrow.

Late tomorrow we will find out which type of leukaemia this is.

There is another family here who were diagnosed on the same day as us last week. I spoke to the mother yesterday and she asked me if I was able to eat. I said yes and she said she wasn't. She had been to the canteen once but told me it was too expensive. In that moment I realised what a wonderful support network we have because I have portioned home-cooked food in my freezer thanks to my neighbour and the constant texts, emails and gifts we receive at the hospital brighten our days no end.

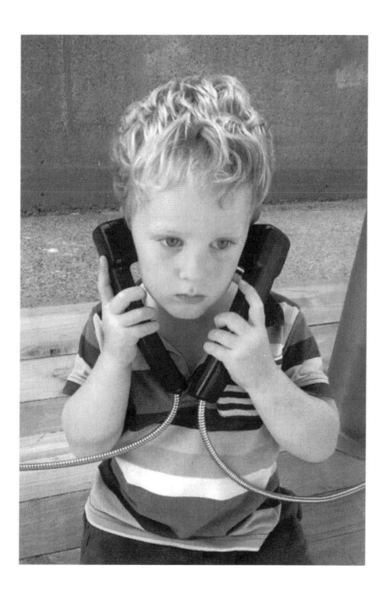

Chapter 2

Regimen A – Induction

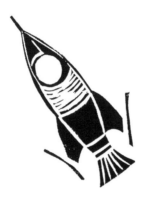

Red blood, yellow night

Blue hospital, white chemo

All Beads of courage

Wednesday, 10th October 2012

Andrew has the commonest and most treatable leukaemia called acute lymphoblastic leukaemia or ALL. The onset is rapid. There is no known cause. I am trying to remember how long he has been symptomatic for. It makes me feel sick to think he has had cancer and I didn't know. I feel so guilty for thinking he was being lazy, but we are eternally grateful to our GP, Dr Navarro, for realising something was wrong and sending us for a blood test straight away. I rang her today to let her know and asked if she had suspected it was leukaemia. She admitted she hadn't suspected it but had known a blood test would show why he was pale and anaemic. Ridiculous to admit it, but I was so relieved when they told us it was leukaemia and not a tumour in his tummy under the spot. They told us not to google the disease as there are a lot of crazy stories and incorrect information on the internet. They have given us print outs from the Macmillan website which is the best and most informative: http://www.macmillan.org.uk/information-and-support/leukaemia/acute-lymphoblastic-all

It was lovely to see Cath this morning. We stood on the pavement outside the house talking. She had been to Primark to pick up some larger size t-shirts for Andrew and was dropping them off. I had taken Clara to school and was then going on to the Royal Marsden. It felt utterly normal to be a Mummy stood on a street corner chatting. Cath is the first person I have spoken in detail to, other than family, since the diagnosis and it was wonderful.

Andrew had a good day as days go. He LOVED the playroom so we played there twice; the Giggle Clowns were there once entertaining the children with squeaky knees and red foam noses: http://uk.theodora.org/en-gb. The playroom has one of those full size rocking horses which Andrew loves to sit on and ride. There is a craft table where he can stick, cut and glue to his heart's content, and another table with moon sand, which is more hygienic than normal sand. The room is well looked after and there are some lovely toys including a wooden hospital and a train set. Since the playroom is opposite the parent's kitchen I can leave Andrew for a moment to refuel on free, strong, milky coffee. He is constantly attached to a fluid drip at the moment, so I have to wheel him around with a stand and plug him in. He likes to stand on the blue metal frame and be wheeled down the corridor. There are lots of plugs in the playroom, so wherever he moves to I can find a plug socket. It is very well designed. He gets into a tangle every now and again with the long Mr Wiggly and has to twist around a few times to free himself.

We are following a protocol called Regimen A using the 2011 ALL guidelines. Tomorrow is 'Day One' of Andrew's treatment, called the Induction Stage, which starts with Dexamethasone (Dex) or steroids; we begin chemotherapy on Day Two.

The steroids will turn him into an emotional little monster apparently. He will have a horrid jab in the leg on Day Four, another general anaesthetic and lumbar puncture on Day Eight and then hopefully he will be home on Day Nine, (next Friday). There was some concern over the possibility of enlarged kidneys; however, Andrew had an ultrasound which showed his kidneys were normal and not enlarged, which is a relief.

The possibility of the leukaemia being in his spinal fluid is less than 1 (this is good). Andrew has learnt to wee in a pot rather than a bed pan, which will make things much easier, especially as Andrew is still being flushed though with fluids. Every time he wees, which is frequently due to the hyper-hydration, I have to come out of the isolation room and take the potty to the sluice room. Here a nurse weighs what he has produced and records it. I then have to wash and sterilise my hands before going back into the isolation room.

The room is cleaned twice a day and the cleaner keeps telling me how much she loves Andrew's hair. I have been thinking, but not saying, how insensitive a comment that is as his hair is surely going to be falling out soon. I don't want to be reminded of how gorgeous his blonde curly locks are; I know they are scrumptious and I don't know what I am going to do or how I am going to feel once they go.

Finally, the ladies in the playroom said we can keep the Imaginext Batcave, as Granddad fixed it and I bought a Batman - they even found a Robin! We have been told going back to school is a possibility for Andrew after four months, but that seems an age away. I cannot believe it has only been a week since we were told Andrew had cancer. It feels so much longer than seven days.

Thursday, October 11th 2012

I didn't go to work today as I have been in hospital with Andrew. The four of us are all together at the hospital. It is very overwhelming having to listen to two children at once. We have had a relaxed day: lots of playing, TV (the

Hong Kong Phooey DVD is a BIG hit) and eating. Clara kept wanting to be near Andrew but, in doing so, she tripped over Mr wiggly and, on one occasion, we feared she was going to pull it out.

Andrew started his liquid oral steroids today and has thrown them up twice. This is particularly stressful and difficult because we have to make him take them again. We are trying small amounts of medicine with loads of ice-cream and Maltesers: anything to disguise the taste. He has to take them twice a day for the next twenty-seven days. We managed one dose eventually, in three stages of about seven millilitres at a time, followed by mouthfuls of Maltesers and ice cream. There were still huge shudders but he was not sick.

I will be dropping off Clara in the morning and then going to work. I cannot believe I have had five years at home and then three weeks into a new job this happens.

Friday, October 12th 2012

Last night that we met our Clic Sargent social worker who said the charity will give us a grant of £170. http://www.clicsargent.org.uk   We can use this for anything we like, but it will more than cover a year's parking at the Royal Marsden. We are now eligible for Disability Benefit for Andrew which means about £74 a week. Again the money will help with travelling costs. Silver linings on a very black cloud. He suggested I don't think about shaving off my hair for charity; I told him I wasn't even thinking about it!

The Clic Sargent social worker gave us two copies of a book called 'Joe has Leukaemia', written from a child's point of view. We won't share it with Andrew yet but it has been a very useful read for us.

I enjoyed going to work and seeing everyone today, though I felt wobbly once I actually got to the office. I cried but it was a relief to talk about it. My boss was fantastic and said to work when I can, in the office or at home if I need to. There is no pressure, which is a huge relief. I feel like I am letting them down so early into a new job. I will try and do one day where I actually leave the house and go to work whilst Joseph 'works from home'. We have a Teaching and Learning Conference next week, so I have been working with colleagues on finalising the primary workshops. I also had a team meeting. It was great to get out of the house and switch my work brain on, but I felt like my head and thought processes were wading through treacle all day.

I picked Clara up from school and felt wobbly all over again, seeing all the other three year olds running around the playground without a care in the world. I did some washing and put the clothes away once she was asleep. Folding up Andrew's clothes made me incredibly sad and I cried for the first time since diagnosis. I've been holding it together by keeping busy, but I miss having him at home. I walked into his empty bedroom and sat and looked around. When I told Mum and Joseph I had cried they were both so pleased and said they had been waiting for it to happen.

Joseph says he and Andrew played for ages with the Imaginex toys. Andrew's phosphates are down, but the doctors are leaving the fluids unchanged for now. Andrew took his medicines mixed into Fromage Frais today, which was more successful. He ate a LOT of food and was sick again.

Saturday, October 13th 2012

I am back in hospital with Andrew. We are now on a ward - Bed One. Has anyone got one of those eye masks they give you on aeroplanes? Andrew took his dexamethasone mixed in Fromage Frais again: no sickness and no shudders. The overeating on steroids has begun; he ate tonnes and made himself sick. He had his first lot of chemo today, called vincristine, through his new portacath, which we call his 'bubble'. The chemotherapy could give Andrew pain in his jaw and achy legs. In the 1950s the poisonous Madagascar periwinkle, or Vinca Rosea, was discovered to have healing properties. Dr JG Armstrong turned the flower into vincristine. We have lots of pink Vinca growing in our garden.

Most of the children on the ward have all sorts of cancers I have not heard of. It is heart-breaking. There are babies who cannot talk to express themselves, so spend a lot of time crying. There is one Year Six girl on our ward who came in after six whole months of going back and forth to the GP. Andrew has cancer, which is devastating, but I am thankful that it is the most curable kind and that he is not too unwell going into treatment. This place makes you realise how much worse it could have been.

On a happier note, one family who were diagnosed four days ahead of us were allowed home today. They walked past the playroom waving, whilst we were playing and had the biggest grins on their faces. Andrew's phosphate levels are more normal, which means less hyper-hydration. So there is a light at the end of the tunnel.

Sunday, October 14th 2012

I had a lovely day at home with Clara, catching up with my brother at Kelsey Park and my daredevil nieces. It is great to be out and about and busy.

Andrew's fluids have been reduced; he wees every three hours or so now. In turn this means more sleep and fewer trips to the sluice room. Joseph is spending a second night at the hospital. This morning Andrew took all three of his medicines, in crushed powder form, mixed with one large spoonful of Fromage Frais. This is a big step forward and better than eighteen millilitres of liquid yuck in syringes. He had a medicine, PEG-asparaginese injected straight into his thigh muscle, like an inoculation, with practically no fuss; he is so used to needles now. He would still prefer to sit in bed watching TV but can be persuaded out into the playroom. I am back at the Royal Marsden tomorrow morning until Tuesday afternoon, so please keep in touch.

Monday, October 15th 2012

It was a bad night last night. Andrew's oxygen levels fell to 91 with anything between 95 and 100 being normal. The nurses spent most of the night fiddling with him, trying to give him oxygen and trying to get a reading on different toes and fingers. Neither Berthoud boy got much sleep. This morning his oxygen level returned to normal again, so the nurses concluded it was because he was 1. Asleep and 2. Lying down and therefore it was nothing to worry about. Yawn.

I am hoping the same does not reoccur tonight. Andrew came off his drip today because all his blood levels are normal. It means he has to drink a lot, about one hundred and fifty millilitres an hour, so I spent most of the day encouraging him to drink a variety of different beverages: apple juice, chocolate milk, Ribena and water. He also needs to eat lots of fruit. The steroids he is on make him hungry, so he over-ate and was sick again. That didn't stop him though, as he just carried on eating his chips. A snack trolley comes around twice a day, morning and afternoon and the children can choose from a selection of crisps and biscuits. Today Andrew ate nine Jaffa cakes.

We have moved to Bed Two on the ward, which is next to a window and is therefore much better, as we have natural light and some fresh air. The two screaming babies have been replaced by two ten-year-old girls, so I am currently listening to EastEnders for the first time in years. Andrew's medicines were mixed with Fromage Frais again today. He will be totally fed up with it by the end of his treatment.

A sparky came yesterday to sort out various electrical jobs in our house and the Sash Window guy is spending the day today fixing Clara and Andrew's windows. I have booked some cleaners to come tomorrow and spend eight hours making our house clean enough for Andrew to come home to. Even the pushchair is booked in for a Glamyourpram clean. Our lovely hairdresser is booked in for tomorrow afternoon. I've invited four giggly girls for a pre-gymnastics play date tomorrow after school. I am organising myself nicely mostly via the internet.

Tuesday, October 16th 2012

Andrew is home!

Andrew slept on the ward from 8pm to 7am. He woke up four times for a wee. I did not sleep well due to a snoring daddy - ears plugs would be useful but then I might not hear the nurses or Andrew if they needed me. Andrew's bloods from last night were normal so we were told, at 9am, that we could come home today. Initially I was thrilled, but the cleaners are not coming until tomorrow and the Sash Window guy is ripping out the windows. I also have those play dates booked, as I thought he was coming out on Friday!

Joseph came back to the Royal Marsden to help pack. There were a lot of people to see and drugs to collect before we left. As we were getting ready to leave one of the play team, asked us if we had collected our beads. I said we hadn't, so she came with the box and showed us what to do. They are called 'beads of courage' and they tell the story of Andrew's treatment through coloured beads, which we thread onto a leather string. Every time he sees a medical professional, has treatment or goes to clinic, he gets a selection of beads.

Black = bloods taken,
White = chemotherapy given,
Blue star = surgery
Red = blood transfusion
Lime = neutropenic
Yellow = a night in hospital

He has given the beads of courage to Clara to look after and will give her the beads every time he collects them from the Royal Marsden; then she will thread them on. We have sixty-two already. By the end of the three years we will have hundreds and hundreds. I have heard that children have a party to celebrate the end of their treatment, where everyone gets together and wraps the beads of courage round them as a thank you: http://www.bechildcanceraware.org/

We left at 3:30pm, updated the car park ticket to a yearly pass, and set off home, like parents bringing their new born baby home for the first time. The house hasn't been cleaned for over two weeks and it was freezing because of the two windows being repaired, so I took Andrew to Mum's. I returned home, popped the heating on, cleaned his room and the bathroom. I collected Andrew who then zonked out in his own bed, probably from sheer relief.

The next four weeks are critical; Andrew is very susceptible to catching infections, which means, in turn, we will end up back in hospital, so we will not be very sociable. The hospital was a cosy, sterile environment and at home I can see and imagine germs everywhere. The next appointment for vincristine chemo is on Friday, so we will be back at the Royal Marsden as daycare patients. For now, I shall enjoy all four of us being at home together under the same roof, and sleeping in my own bed.

Wednesday, October 17th 2012
Day one at home – two weeks since diagnosis.

Andrew slept better last night compared to being in the hospital. However, he is used to having one or other of us asleep next to him. I ended up on a make shift bed on his floor, so much for sleeping in my own bed. The sash window company came back at 8am to do Andrew's room. We had to empty it entirely to prevent his furniture and toys from being covered in dust, so much for a lie in. The hospital warned us against building work because of the mould spores which could be released.

We all took Clara to school which was lovely and felt 'normal', though I was quite paranoid about people and their germs not getting too close to Andrew. I enjoyed Clara's Harvest Festival celebration in the local church; it brought a few tears to my eyes, especially when I walked to the hall where Andrew's preschool runs. I haven't spoken to them about what has happened. The headteacher gave me a big hug and we both had a little cry. They are going to keep Andrew's place open so he can go back eventually.

Andrew had his gorgeous blond curls cut short today, necessary to prepare us all for when his hair falls out. He cried and said it hurt. His head is very sensitive. He took his medicine this morning, mixed with Nutella, and this evening, mixed in chocolate Angel Delight with some party bag treats. He couldn't go to a friend's party but was still given the party bag. He was sick twice. We need to work out why he is being sick, as I don't want him to have anti-sickness drugs too. He gets cold easily so the heating is on all the time. He drank more than the required thousand millilitres of liquid though, so is hydrated. Bed time was very peaceful; Clara read a few poems from her christening book. She has been very kind, giving Andrew cuddles, telling him she loves him and playing Guess Who patiently. We had a yummy casserole for dinner, thanks to Cath. I am looking forward to a glass of wine and a cake, thanks to other friends. You are a fabulous bunch of people and we truly could not do this or be as strong as we are without you all.

Thursday, October 18th 2012
Day Two at home.

Today has been one of the hardest days. Joseph's uncle died last week so he has been to Wiltshire for the funeral with the family. I have been on my own with Andrew. He is constantly hungry. To try and combat the sickness, we decided we would give him small amounts to eat and often, so I fed him every hour. He wanted scrambled egg on toast, beans on toast (twice), a brioche, biscuits, a fruit kebab, cucumber and cakes. He eats but, two minutes later, says he is hungry and wants more, so I spend the next hour fobbing off requests for food. With every food prepared, the kitchen has to be cleaned, new plates and cutlery used and worktops sprayed with anti-bacterial cleaner so as not to create germs. I have to wash my hands thoroughly with soap and water. I have eczema on my hands, so they are getting dry and sore. Every time I wash them I put cream on to moisturise, but then I have to wash them again; it is frustrating and my hands are cracked and painful. I have been using the hand sanitizer the Royal Marsden gave us a lot too but it makes the cuts sting.

I ate breakfast at 10:30am and lunch at 2pm (all in secret). If Andrew smells food or hears someone talking about it he wants it NOW, and has no concept of the time it takes to cook. All was going relatively swimmingly until Clara wanted pizza at dinner time. Andrew had some too but was sick, as he doesn't chew pizza and it had greasy pepperoni oil on it. I think greasy food makes him sick, and orange juice too, which is too acidic for his sensitive stomach. I feel drained from the constant attention he demands and am trying to balance it with unpacking, getting jobs done, worrying about germs and giving Clara the attention she deserves too.

The community nurses came today and gave me a sharps bin and a whole bunch of medical equipment for when they come to access his port weekly. Suddenly the enormity of it all is hitting home: we are only on Day Eight of a three-year programme of chemotherapy. Treatment is three years for boys (and two years for girls) as the cancerous blast cells could hide in the testicles and they cannot be treated directly. The extra year is needed to make sure the leukaemia cells have gone from there too. He will be in seven and in Year Two when this is all over.

Friday, 19th October 2012
Day Three at home.

Andrew had a MUCH better day. First of all, there has been NO SICKNESS (so far); we let him eat more in one sitting, and helped him understand that when his tummy hurts it means he is full, not that he is going to be sick. He still asked for food in between meals but with less ferocity.

We took Andrew out this morning to get some fresh air and a new football from the toy shop: nice and normal, but it was stressful hoping that no one would cough over him. I put the rain cover over him, which he hated, but at least he was safe in a protected bubble. We were back at the Royal Marsden this afternoon for his third vincristine chemo. This was the first time his portacath had been accessed. A needle was inserted through his skin and into the portacath with a wiggly line for bloods to be taken and chemotherapy medicine to be put in. We have been dreading it, expecting him to scream and shout as he had with the cannulas. The nurse thought he had magic cream (Ametop) on, to numb the area, but he didn't, so we opted for the much quicker cold spray to numb the area instead.

The Steri-Strips on the scar, where doctors had inserted the port, were removed and the area was cleaned with a 'magic wand.' Joseph held Andrew to keep his arms out of the way. Andrew hates having his arms held, but it is important he doesn't make any sudden movements. The nurse inserted the needle; blood came out, and chemotherapy went in, whilst I blew bubbles like crazy to distract Andrew. Then he was deaccessed and the line was removed. It was all done in twenty minutes. Andrew said "that didn't hurt", which was such a relief. His platelet levels are low, at nineteen, but not low enough to require a transfusion over the weekend. Another day done, thanks to all of you.

Saturday, October 20th 2012

Another day of no sickness (yet). Andrew is totally off anything sweet, is mainly eating bread products and is still obsessed with eggs and ketchup. When he starts shivering, we know he needs to drink more. His tummy hurts today, mainly due to the vincristine chemo yesterday, but he flips flops between thinking he is hungry, needing a wee or saying he is about to be sick. He is displaying lots of terrible two behaviours and is exhausting to manage; Joseph is so much better than me at distracting him and engaging him in play. Joseph and Clara swam in the deep pool at the spa, whilst Andrew and I napped. Tonight's job is filling in the Disability Living Allowance (DLA) Benefit form and buying a new washing machine and tumble dryer. It is not great timing that ours have both packed up as Andrew is frequently sick. Mum came to the rescue, doing all the loads of washing for us today. We have got the DLA guidance from CLIC Sargent, which makes the form so much easier to fill in, but it still takes hours and I can't claim any money for three months anyway. I cannot believe my son is going to be registered disabled.

Monday, 22nd October 2012

Every year in the run up to Christmas, as an Usborne Books at home rep, I do a big book order. This year I will be doing the same; however, all the books will be commission free (-24%). I hope some of you may choose to buy a book or two as the more bought means the more in free books Usborne give to me. I will donate these free books to the Royal Marsden in Sutton, the hospital that has been, is and will be looking after Andrew in his cancer treatment: www.usborne.com. The Marsden have a book box, so I am planning to buy them some Usborne stencils for the art and crafts table, noisy button books for younger children to enjoy, and a few chapter books for the older children.

Tuesday, 23rd October 2012

Andrew had his first bloods taken today by the community nurses at home. He was very fearful but eventually sat still whilst she accessed his port, took the bloods and deaccessed him again. He sits on my lap and I have to pretend not to hold his arms out of the way, whilst actually being ready to grab him should he try and move as the needle goes in. Afterwards he said "it didn't hurt", so the fear is all in his head. The bloods showed, as we suspected because he is pale, that he needs a platelet transfusion tomorrow at Queen Elizabeth, Woolwich so he is 'well' for his general anaesthetic on Thursday and vincristine chemo on Friday. The nurse who rang me with the blood results was called Alison and is a mum at Andrew's preschool. I did not realise she was an oncology nurse - small world. Platelets take about thirty minutes to transfuse, so nowhere near as long as the four hours needed for a bag of blood, and we are warned he could develop a rash. He has had two platelet transfusions before with no adverse reactions but seeing as each bag comes from someone different, you don't know what might happen.

Thursday, 25th October 2012

It has been a tough couple of days emotionally. Yesterday there was a lot of waiting around for the platelet transfusion and Andrew got tired and anxious. We had to be at the Royal Marsden for 8:15am this morning. Andrew was nil by mouth from 4am so he was VERY hungry, and VERY grumpy and VERY much wanting a ham sandwich every two minutes between 7:30am and midday when he finally set off for his operation.

I didn't realise there is an operation room in the daycare part of the hospital. I thought we would be going upstairs again to where he had his first operation. The anaesthetic was given very swiftly and it surprised me when I saw his eyes roll back, and hearing him whimper as he fell asleep was horrible. The lumbar puncture lasted only twelve minutes and then he was back, eating chips and ham sandwiches. I only just had enough time to run for a coffee at the café and recover from seeing him being put under.

I didn't know we had to wait for an hour to check he was okay, so we finally got home at 2pm, having left at 7:15am. He found sitting in the car uncomfortable, so I need to find something for him to put his legs on; having them dangle makes them ache. He has slept for an hour on the sofa and now I am cooking him pasta with sauce, frankfurters and peas. I am off to work tomorrow whilst Joseph takes him back again for vincristine chemo, which should hopefully be quicker.

At 4:34pm
Andrew has a temperature, so is back off to the hospital, this time to our (not very) local Queen Elizabeth Hospital in Woolwich. He is neutropenic, which means he has no white blood cells to fight infection. They will probably give him some antibiotics. He will also have to be accessed again – I wish we had left the wiggly in earlier, although I didn't know he was going to get a temperature.

At 9:43pm
Andrew's temperature has come back down. He is on intravenous (IV) antibiotics and will still have his vincristine chemo and will be home on Sunday at the earliest.
Do me a favour, if you have critical illness cover on your mortgage, please check it also includes your children, because you might then get a lump sum too. Our policy doesn't include the children - we have not lost anything,

but you don't know what is around the corner and it might be best to check.

Friday, 26th October 2012

Andrew is still 'well' in hospital. He slept most of the day and the temperature has not returned so we still hope he will be out on Sunday morning; if not, he will be ambulanced to the Royal Marsden on Monday for his vincristine chemo. I worked today at the Teaching and Learning conference, so I had to be up at 5:30am, but I woke at 4am. I couldn't sleep; my head was buzzing. I am fit for nothing this evening so am going to bed at the same time as Clara. At least it is half term now. It is my turn to do a shift in hospital tomorrow - keep in touch.

Saturday, October 27th 2012

It is 9:15pm and a three-hour blood transfusion has started. Andrew will have observations every fifteen minutes. It is going to be a long night.

Sunday, October 28th 2012

We are all home, exhausted, but home again.

Monday, October 29th 2012

Any more book orders? We are £18 away from £600 worth of books which means we receive 60% of the total raised in free books for the Marsden - WOW! I spoke to playroom team about the order today and they will use the books as presents for children who are on the ward on their birthday or at Christmas, as well as restocking the book corner. Wonderful.

Andrew has lots of issues at the moment, including high blood pressure and a hurty tummy, so we have new medicines. I'm hoping to sort it out, but it all pales into insignificance when I know what the emergency alarms at the Royal Marsden meant for one family today.

Tuesday, October 30th 2012
I am having a lovely birthday. Thank you for all the messages, cards and texts. Thanks for all the lovely presents that make me feel thoroughly spoilt and a little bit more like me again. Thanks for my pummelling massage, which was so needed, and to Michelle for allowing me to book another one. Most of all, thanks to Joseph for thinking I am Wonder Woman and treating me as such all day. Off out tonight to see Skyfall whilst my mum holds the fort.

Wednesday, 31st October 2012
We have raised £550 in free books for the Royal Marsden children! Thank you!

Thursday, November 1st 2012
Andrew has a sore bottom. It is one of the known side effects of his high blood pressure medication. It is irritating his gut, but it is needed to counter the side effects of his steroids while he is having chemotherapy.

So far this morning Andrew has eaten eleven homemade scotch pancakes and three selection boxes of Kellogg's cereal AND has not been sick.

Friday, November 2nd 2012
Another day on my own with both children; so far so good: one is watching TV and one is on the IPad. It will be

interesting to see what Clara thinks when she sees Andrew have bloods taken later, as I have booked her and me in for a flu jab tomorrow. We are all eligible for a flu jab now, as we have to keep well to ensure Andrew does not catch the flu. Andrew woke up five times in the night but is not needing us to sleep on his bedroom floor anymore, so there is some progress being made.

Andrew's blood results from today show he is repairing his body himself. His platelet levels have risen but not because he has had a transfusion. The same is true with his HB level and, for the first time, his neutrophil levels are over one - this is all GOOD news.

Sunday, November 4th 2012
I feel achy, but I was injected with flu yesterday. I hope Clara feels OK and I don't feel any worse; I am not sure I can do this knackered AND ill. Does anyone have a baby monitor lurking unused which we could borrow for a bit? It would be useful to have so we can hear if Andrew needs us when we are downstairs. He got upset last night, as he was calling for us when we were watching TV.

Monday, November 5th 2012
We spent the afternoon at the Royal Marsden for vincristine chemo, but came away not having had it in the end. They were concerned about Andrew's distended tummy and shallow breathing. They prodded and poked, three consultants came to look. He had an x-ray and gave a urine sample. The outcome was that he is FULL of poo; his small and large intestine are blocked, so he has to drink Movical to get moving in time for chemo on Wednesday. His glucose blood level is high, another side effect of the

dexamethasone, and if he had had ketones in his urine we would have been admitted, but thankfully there were none. We have been given Movical to use rather than Lactulose, which was making his constipation worse.

We have to monitor his blood sugar levels by pin prick test four times a day because he may end up having to have insulin if it does not drop. His blood pressure is up again and so the medication for this has also been increased. Roll on the end of the steroids on 14th November. The doctor did not give me a pin prick machine but told me the community nurses could find one for me. The nurses told me they didn't have such machines and the Royal Marsden should have given me one. I ended up scouring the internet and buying one myself. I am sure I can sell it on EBAY eventually.

Tuesday, November 6th 2012

Andrew's bowels are on the move with LOTS of screaming. Bless him, and now he is back in bed. We are very proud of him, as he has swallowed his steroid tablets whole, so there is no more need to crush them and hide them in something to disguise the taste. He has never been great at chewing food. When he is sick, whole pieces of pasta come back up, so we thought we would try getting him to swallow tablets by practising with mini smarties. However, Joseph tried with one of the steroid tablets first and he managed it!

Wednesday, November 7th 2012

We had a fairly quick trip to the Royal Marsden today: in and out in two hours. The consultant was pleased the Movical had been working. Andrew's blood sugar levels were 4.7, 6.2 and 7.1, which means we don't have to finger prick him at home anymore and, more importantly, there is no need for insulin.

His blood pressure is still a bit high at 122/78 but they decided to give the new medication a while to work before making another change. He had his vincristine through his port and we have to be back in the morning at 7:45am for another lumbar puncture. This means another nil by mouth on dexamethasone but the last one for a while. Tomorrow we will start reducing his steroids, so all the side effects - high blood pressure, high glucose levels, constant hunger, wakefulness, feebleness, constipation, low mood and lethargy - will hopefully start to drift away.

His blood results continue to climb too. The next month involves Mercaptopurine (6mp) chemo, taken orally at home, and regular lumbar punctures, but everyone says the first month is the worst and we are nearly at the end.

Thursday, November 8th 2012
Shattered.com – I am looking forward to work tomorrow to have a break from being the main carer.

Friday, 9th November 2012
Another day at work in the office with a lot of paperwork and systems to be put into place: just my cup of tea.

Saturday, November 10th 2012
I am looking forward to, but feeling a bit guilty about, a day in London with the very lovely Sacha and Jane. It will be my second day in a row of not being the main carer. I am looking forward to another delicious lunch at Jamie's

Italian and a girly gossip whilst shopping around Covent Garden. When I get home tonight we will enjoy some fireworks and eat curry whilst watching Louis Smith dance on Strictly Come Dancing.

Sunday, November 11th 2012

Andrew's chronic constipation is so hard to manage. If he has too much Movical he gets the runs; too little and he moans in pain as he did tonight. Of course it is also a balance with the food he eats and the other medication he is taking. We are not allowed to give him ibuprofen or paracetamol for the pain. We have codeine, which we could give him, but this also makes him constipated. Joseph likens what we are going through to someone turning up and giving us a newborn baby unannounced. We have sleep deprivation and don't know what the infant needs or wants, but we still have to work, run the house, entertain a toddler, and take care of a five-year-old who is functioning at four times the speed of Andrew. We have been pressganged into the cancer world. Fingers crossed Andrew settles and we manage to get some sleep, albeit in shifts tonight. It is my turn to sleep first.

Monday, November 12th 2012

When Andrew was diagnosed with leukaemia we were told he was eligible for Disability Living Allowance and a Blue Badge for the car. Both seemed like extra financial perks at the time. Now however Andrew cannot even stand without support let alone walk anywhere. He cannot climb stairs, sit up unaided, roll over in bed or lift his arms and legs to get dressed without us; the cancer is disabling and the Blue Badge will be a blessing. In the meantime, we make him use his legs to walk to the loo. If we don't do this, he will have other problems in the long run, but mainly we carry him (all twenty kilograms of him). It is my lower back that suffers the most; hot baths and massages keep the pain in check, and the odd day at work gives my body a break from the constant weight-lifting.

I think being diagnosed with ALL at three years old is another silver lining on the black cloud of caner because Andrew doesn't know what he is missing out on e.g. swimming lessons and pre-school. It must be a lot harder with a child who is older. Andrew has no concentration span for much other than TV and not even for that sometimes; I cannot imagine trying to get him to do school work.

Cancer mummies: Morning all. So we have finished our first month and are nearing the end of the steroids. We have started taking oral mercaptopurine chemo at home. Could anyone give me a heads up for what to expect next e.g. weight loss, not eating, more energy, more sleep, less sleep? Everyone says the first month is the hardest. I am kind of hoping this is the case and everything lets up a little!

> *Hi Melody,*
> *Great stuff! You are over the first month. As you know, my son also has ALL and we're just a little ahead of you at three and half months, and about to finish interim maintenance. We certainly found a big difference in Month Two; he had much more energy, lost his steroid weight gain and had fewer hospital visits. In fact, we visited Leeds Castle at three and a half weeks into treatment and he*

*hadn't the energy to even go to the play area,
never mind walk. A week and a half later, he
ran all over the place; it was such a massive
difference!*

Tuesday, November 13th 2012

Back from our first trip of the week to the Royal Marsden.
We met with our consultant today. He seemed pleased
with Andrew's progress; everything is 'normal', such as the
loss of mobility and lack of sleep. The BIG result, which
determines if we swap onto Regimen C, which is more
aggressive, was not back, so we have to wait until the end
of the week. The next consultant appointment is in nine
weeks' time in January 2013.

We discussed whether there was a benefit in switching to
private treatment using our medical insurance but were
told there is not. The best paediatric oncology is via the
NHS. We also discussed why we couldn't use the Royal
Marsden as our local as it was equidistant to our house
compared to the Queen Elizabeth. I didn't realise the
Royal Marsden wasn't used by anyone as a local: the use
of their beds is booked in advance so you cannot turn up
uninvited. That is what the local is for – emergency care.
There are no other locals near us, so we have to stay with
the Queen Elizabeth.

We met occupational therapy to ask if we could borrow
a Major McLaren Pushchair whilst Andrew isn't walking.
They gave me a secondhand one straight away and told
me to apply for a new through the wheelchair service in
Bromley.

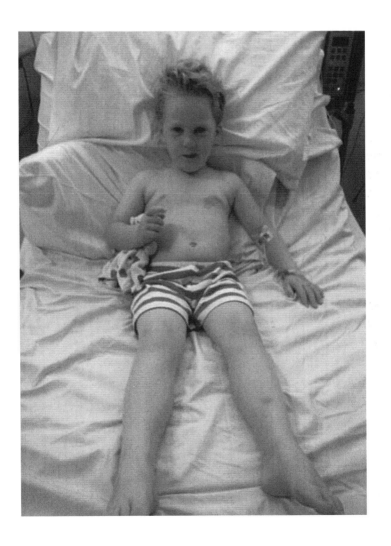

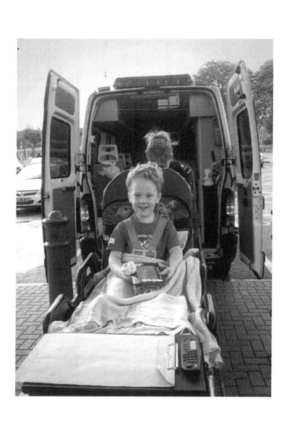

Chapter 3

Regimen A - Consolidation

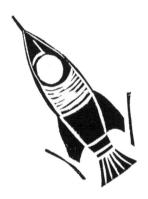

We slept with dry food

By our bed for the sickness

Cheerios were best

Thursday, 15th November 2012

Andrew has started the next stage of treatment called Consolidation. Joseph is with him at the Royal Marsden today for a lumbar puncture where intrathecal methotrexate will be injected into his spine. These lumbar punctures will be weekly now. I will be back with Andrew on Friday for an echocardiogram (ECG) of his heart. We have to give Andrew a chemotherapy drug called mercaptopurine every day at home – an hour after he eats his last meal.

I travelled to work today by commuting up the Victoria Line to Seven Sisters to support a newly-qualified teacher in her class. It was nice to have time to sit and do nothing on the tube other than read a novel.

Andrew had his first bath in six weeks, which he enjoyed; he actually lay down in it. You can see how thin his hair is in the water and, on washing it, more is falling out. We had lovely feedback from Clara's teacher at Parent's Evening. We are very proud of her. I think it is a credit to her and the school that, over the last six weeks, she has continued to learn, grow and be a delight.

Friday, 16th November 2012

Cancer mummies: How does being neutropenic work? Andrew was but now isn't (11.2): will he be again? Is it related to a particular drug or a round of treatment or is it random?

If Andrew is having chemotherapy, then it kills all of his white cells and the neutrophils which they contain. This means that his immune system is severely compromised and he is unable to fight off infection. This is why patients have to go straight to hospital if they spike a temperature of thirty-eight degrees or more. A two or three day course of IV antibiotics can be transfused to take the place of the depleted immune system. A week after chemotherapy ends, the bone marrow is able to function normally again and produce HB, platelets, white blood cells and neutrophils.

You might find there is a pattern to it or it might be random. My son was often neutropenic in the first few months and we were in and out of hospital with infections, but you can be neutropenic and not pick anything up. He is now in maintenance and hasn't been neutropenic once, but his neutrophils go sky high when he is on dex (he has one dose of vincristine and then dex for five days) and then they go down and down until the following month when the dex boosts them up again. Our kids have so many drugs and each has different side effects, so it is very difficult to predict but you get to know your own child's pattern to an extent.

It is the job of the chemotherapy to keep his immune system supressed, so if everything is low then you know the chemotherapy is working.

Sunday, November 18th 2012

Andrew's steroid fog seems to be lifting; he is telling jokes and even being a bit cheeky! His mobility has yet to return but hopefully it will. He is waking less in the night, so Joseph and I are having crazy dreams, as we are sleeping longer and deeper than we have in weeks. We had an autumn leaf fight in the park yesterday. Simple delights.

The house got too hot last night, so Andrew overheated and was 0.3 of a degree away from having to go to the local hospital for a forty-eight hour stay. If he gets a temperature of thirty-eight degrees we have to wait half an hour and retake his temperature. If it is still high, we have to go into the local. If it reaches thirty-eight point five degrees we have to drop everything, day or night, and go straight in. Luckily with the heating off and a window open his temperature has returned to normal.

Monday, November 19th 2012

Slow improvements continue. Andrew has been walking more today but, like a new walker, needs a hand to hold and tires quickly. If there is a step, his legs tend to go from under him too, so he cannot be left on his own to walk. He has played today for a sustained amount of time... jigsaws! He can sit on the floor and complete them, so they are a perfect toy for now. We have also watched the fight scenes from Kung Fu Panda a couple of times, as it is his new favourite film. Having eaten constantly for thirty-five days his appetite has dropped. He eats lots for breakfast, then it tapers off for the rest of the day. He also does not know what he wants to eat. I find myself cooking food he thinks he wants but then doesn't, so he gets cross.

I am finding the best way to appease him is to present him with a buffet of foods and then pretend to eat them myself; he will tuck in. This is not a helpful strategy for my attempts at weight loss though. He also doesn't want to do anything which reminds him of his previous life, like going to the park or thinking about preschool. I suppose it must be very strange for him to understand what is going on.

Tuesday, November 20th 2012

To remind me to take nothing for granted, the local hospital has phoned to say Andrew's blood results from this morning show he is neutropenic and will need a thirty minute platelet transfusion soon. He needs a three-hour blood transfusion NOW, so off to the Queen Elizabeth in Woolwich we go.

Wednesday, November 21st 2012

We have had a lovely day. Granny, and her golden retriever Kesia, arrived with a new toy for the children, a remote control car. Andrew can stand now to control the car then shuffles to chase after it. A perfectly timed present. The Beckenham Round Table have also granted us some money to buy Andrew a much-needed new bed with truckle, so we can all get a more comfortable night's sleep. I filled in their application form and one of the members rang me today. The committee had met and unanimously decided we can have the money. How wonderful and what a relief! One or other of us still ends up on his bedroom floor most nights. If you attended the Fireworks in the Recreation Ground this year thank you for adding to the charity's profits, which in turn go to helping people like us: http://www.roundtable.co.uk/

Thursday, November 22nd 2012

Joseph took Andrew to the Royal Marsden today for his weekly lumbar puncture whilst I journeyed to work on the Victoria Line to support another newly-qualified teacher. It is so important for my sanity to be able to escape the pressures of being at home with Andrew; to go to work, have a break and have time thinking about something completely different.

Saturday, November 24th 2012

I had a tough night with Andrew and a hurting tummy; he didn't settle until 4am. He has been sick three times this morning so we are back at the Queen Elizabeth in Woolwich, having him checked over. They don't seem too worried, especially as he has no temperature and is playing on the Nintendo Wii whilst eating babybel and Coco Pops! Hopefully if we can get him to have his medicine and keep it down we can go home.

Monday, November 26th 2012

A fairly normal day today; I took boxes to the tip, urine samples to Woolwich Hospital, did a spot of shopping in Bromley and had lunch with Cath. We came home for a nap and then had playdates for Clara and Andrew. It was so nice to see Andrew playing with toys and interacting with friends again. I know it may not last but I am appreciating it whilst it does. It is not the same 'normal' of a few months ago, before he was diagnosed, but I will take anything that feels like normal now and hold onto it tightly. Bloods are being taken in the morning by the community team, so fingers crossed it does not mean another trip to hospital like last week.

Tuesday, November 27th 2012

Andrew woke up ONCE last night. He would wake in the night even before the cancer, so I cannot ask for more than that.

Wednesday, November 28th 2012

I left at 6:45am this morning to go to Tottenham and help out with a practice inspection at a school. I got home at 7:30pm to Andrew who had twisted his ankle and had needed to go to the Princess Royal University Hospital to be checked out. Thankfully he was already home and there was nothing wrong. One of the joys of taking a child with cancer to A&E is that the triage is fast! Andrew did not wake at all last night, so I had to check he was still breathing before I left this morning. I am always worrying. We are off to the Royal Marsden in the morning for an 8:15am lumbar puncture and general anaesthetic and will hopefully be told the news we have been waiting for about his MRD results.

Thursday, November 29th 2012

The results of the Day Twenty Eight Minimal Residual Disease (MRD) are in and Andrew still has a trace of residual leukaemia cells in his blood, which means they found traces of the original cancerous cells. He is in remission now but needs the more intensive chemotherapy regimen to ensure the trace cells are killed and do not regrow, causing a relapse. These results mean he would be 'high risk' for a relapse if we were to continue as we were. We are not upset as we have been discussing the possible options and had decided the more intensive regimen would be a good scenario – none of what we are going through is pleasant, so why not do a little bit more to ensure it stays away.

In reality it means weekly trips to the Royal Marsden plus daily visits from the community nurses, so Andrew will have to be accessed most of the time. There are no new medicines to be taken at home which is a relief. Our trips to the Royal Marsden are scheduled to be on the next five Mondays, including Christmas Eve and New Year's Eve.

I am so pleased not to have any more lumbar punctures in the next eight weeks. I hope there is not another load of side effects to cope with and I am worried about him feeling sick. Andrew is a lot perkier, walking more, and is generally happier and sleeping. I hope that does not deteriorate too. It is a shame our appointments are on Mondays so there will be no more Berthoud/Perrott days of fun for a while.

Cath Perrott and I met each other in 2007 at NCT birthing classes. As the babies turned one and mum's in the group returned to work Cath and I continued to see each other weekly. We met up for toddler classes and then play dates. I refer to Cath as my 'Monday' friend as seeing her, Lucas and Laila every Monday is, or was, a highlight of my week.

Sunday, December 2nd 2012

We had a lazy morning followed by a mummy and daughter trip to the London Aquarium and cake, then home for Strictly Come Dancing on catch up. Andrew is walking a lot more, albeit jerkily, and even climbed into bed tonight and started waving his legs around saying "I'm cycling". I am anxious about the coming weeks and what it will mean for him and us. Fingers crossed for minimal side effects please.

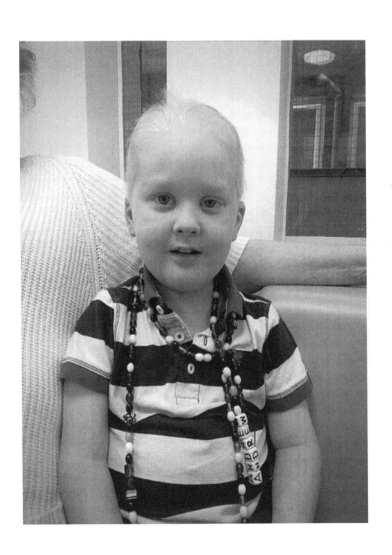

Chapter 4

Regimen C – Augmented
Consolidation - Part 1

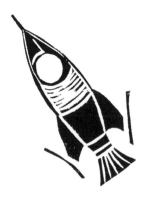

Delays, frustration

Patience is a virtue when

Sitting and waiting

Monday, December 3rd 2012

Two months have passed since Andrew's diagnosis; we have thirty-four months to go. It has been lovely to meet people in the hospital and hear what the path is like for them, but sometimes too much information is not useful, as it makes me worry. Andrew has automatically been put onto an anti-sickness medication called ondansetron because of the new cyclophosphamide chemo drug given today. One mum I met said her son did one big vomit every day but did not feel nauseous all the time. Andrew threw up today at about 7:30pm, so maybe he will be the same.

Other Mums in the online support groups say they have spent some time in their local hospital every week as this cytarabine chemo causes a rise in temperature. It also causes low white blood count and low neutrophil levels, which in turn can cause fever and infection, so we expect to have some visits to our local hospital in the next eight weeks. We knew it would be hard again and I am back to thinking about each hour and day as it comes.

Tuesday, December 4th 2012

I am having a half hour at the pool, watching Clara swim, to have a break from a truly awful afternoon. The new drug is causing Andrew leg pain, tummy pain, sickness, nausea, grumpiness, and tiredness, loss of appetite and sore eyes. He didn't know what he wanted this afternoon. He wanted a cuddle but it hurt, to be left alone but not, to lie down but it hurt, to sit but not; all his frustration came out through hitting me every time we had a cuddle and then massive tantrums when he was cross with himself for hitting me. I couldn't get him in the pushchair to get Clara at 3:30pm so I ended up carrying him and hurt my back, he basically cried from 2pm until 6pm almost nonstop. Everything feels relentless at the moment. We had a bad night last night so fingers crossed we can get some sleep tonight. At least I have two days at work now.

Wednesday, December 5th 2012

Joseph looked after Andrew today whilst I travelled to work on the Victoria Line to Tottenham and spent time in class with more newly-qualified teachers. Andrew napped on and off. He did not complain of nausea all day, until 7:30pm, when again he was sick. Not much came out this time as he had not eaten or drunk much. He didn't watch TV all day, so there were no big tantrums or mood swings when we turned it off, which is good. It was lovely that Andrew wanted to go into the playroom and play a game with me when I got home. There is not much need for movicol at the moment because the new cytarabine chemo (third dose today; last one for the week tomorrow) has given him an upset tummy, so all in all, a slight improvement on my day with him yesterday, even though new hurdles have been put up. Fingers crossed, please, for some sleep tonight for Joseph who is on 'duty'.

10:05pm

Andrew and Joseph are off to hospital as Andrew has a temperature of 38.5 degrees. So much for getting a good night's sleep.

Thursday, December 6th 2012 Mum came to the rescue and took Clara to school this morning, so I could go to work in Peckham. I am now in the hospital with Andrew so Joseph can be at home and go to work tomorrow. Andrew's temperature is down, as is his heart rate, after

Calpol and two strong antibiotics overnight. He has thrush on the roof of his mouth and one ulcer on his bottom left gum. He is not constipated but is very dehydrated so is also on a fluid drip. The blood results suggest he has got an infection of some kind, but we won't know exactly what until tonight or tomorrow. It is probably gastro-related due to the vomiting and diarrhoea. Mum has arranged for all our carpets to be cleaned whilst we are in hospital due to the number of times Andrew has been sick upstairs and because he had a few 'accidents' on the playroom carpets downstairs too.

Friday, December 7th 2012

Andrew had a disturbed night and was up every hour between 7pm and midnight. He needed Calpol for the temperatures and codeine for the pain but finally settled and slept until 6am when he was woken for his morning IV antibiotics. He has come off the IV fluid drip so again has to drink lots and lots. There has been no sickness, but there are still some problems at the other end. He is due a blood transfusion today as his haemoglobin (HB) is 6.7. His temperature is currently normal, which is great. We are still waiting for the forty-eight-hour blood culture results, which will tell us what kind of virus or infection he has. His hair is falling out thick and fast now too. It is all over his pillow and keeps ending up in his food; cutting his hair short was not a great idea because it is harder to pick out of bowls of cereal.

Saturday, December 8th 2012

Andrew has an infection in his gut called C. diff, which is very contagious, so we are in isolation here at the Queen Elizabeth. He has started a ten-day course of antibiotics which will hopefully get rid of it, but he may always carry it now in his gut therefore it may continue to rear up. He can have his last cytarabine chemo of the week today, though the one we have is out of date so we are hoping the Royal Marsden can make us a new one and send it over. As long as the diarrhoea and temperature remain under control we can come home in the morning.

He slept badly last night - awake every hour, moaning, weeing, pooing (green liquid - not nice) or being fiddled with by a nurse. He was so upset at about 1am that we had to watch some Cbeebies on the laptop to stop him from screaming. He has eaten today: a brioche, dry cheerios, Maltesers and chocolate cornflake cakes so far. He had a blood transfusion yesterday afternoon, as his levels were down to 6.7, but the levels are only up to 8.0 today which still seems low to me. We are back at the Royal Marsden on Monday for Week Two of the cytarabine as normal.

Sunday, December 9th 2012
The most special part of picking our Christmas tree today is that Andrew is home from hospital to help decorate it, (though actually he is in bed asleep).

Monday, December 10th 2012
A quick trip to the Royal Marsden has turned into a seven-day stint in isolation for a course of antibiotics. We have to stay at the Royal Marsden tonight, but we will go to the Queen Elizabeth in Woolwich when they have a bed for us. Every cloud has a silver lining though, as Father Christmas happened to be visiting the Royal Marsden today, so he waved at Andrew through the door in isolation and gave

him a present. I rushed after him to tell him what Andrew wanted in his stocking.

Tuesday, December 11th 2012

A strange day with lots of sickness and poo. I have been persuading Andrew to take drugs and persuading him to eat and to drink. His temperature has gone up and down all day. He is now having more blood; the transfusion is due to end at 11pm. I have been out of the room three times only to make coffee. We have entertained ourselves with YouTube, the TV, the IPad and the Cbeebies website. Thank goodness for the Lego advent calendar I bought too. The play team kept popping in to give us crafts to do: make a card, colour in a shepherd, make a Father Christmas house or pipe cleaner wreaths. We are still at the Royal Marsden, but should be going to the Queen Elizabeth in Woolwich by ambulance tomorrow if they have a room. We are quite comfy here for now. I would rather stay here.

Wednesday, December 12th 2012

Apparently the C. diff is not causing Andrew's temperature and nothing else is showing up in his blood cultures, so it is probably the cytarabine which is the culprit. Today he had the cytarabine with an antihistamine, as he might be having an allergic reaction. Fingers crossed that this is what it is and the antihistamine will stop his temperature from spiking again - so far so good. We have one more cytarabine tomorrow, then we have a much needed break for two weeks. We have vincristine chemo before we start another two weeks of cytarabine on New Year's Eve. We may well be spending the first two weeks of 2013 in hospital too.

1:42pm

There is a room at our local hospital, Queen Elizabeth in Woolwich, now so I am loading up on snacks and craft activities to take with us. There is an intermittent TV signal and no Wi-Fi there. If anyone local has some different DVDs we could watch, I would be grateful.

The dietician has planted the seed by saying it is rare for someone on regimen C to get through without needing a nasogastric feeding tube (NG tube) down his nose – this may be likely but short term and hopefully not for a while. Please will Andrew to drink, eat and get better so we can go home. I don't want him to have an NG tube. The antibiotics finish on Monday so we won't be home before then.

Thursday, December 13th 2012

Andrew had a temperature of 39.9 this morning but has had nothing since the cytarabine chemo. He managed a few spoonfuls of Coco Pops, but not much else, and is still drinking his fluids. He actually slept well last night and I was only woken three or four times. The set up here is ridiculous - we are in a room with no en-suite loo. Remember, we are in isolation for a gut infection, so he either has to leave the room to go to the loo, or go in a bed pan, which I then have to take out to deposit.

The aerials do not work, so every room has a television with no access to channels. I brought in an aerial from home and have rigged it up to get our TV to work. There are only four rooms in oncology here, but we don't have our own kitchen to prepare hot drinks or meals for us. We have to go to the children's ward and risk walking past infectious children. There is talk of turning one of the two bathrooms into a kitchen, but when it will actually happen I don't know. There is a fridge in the playroom, so at least we can keep food in there.

Andrew had an ultrasound today, to look at his gut; it looks like his small intestine is inflamed, which might explain all the issues he has been having. We are now halfway through the week of antibiotics. I have until 7pm tomorrow, then I am set free. Andrew wants to go home so is very grumpy with everyone. He is asleep again, thanks to the codeine, so is peaceful at the moment.

I popped out for a few hours to see Clara's nativity. I haven't seen her all week, so I felt desperately sad when I saw her as a beautiful angel on the stage. It was heartbreaking because I knew I had to go back to the hospital again and I have missed her so much. I cried silently all the way through. Afterwards the teachers let me have a cuddle with her in the medical room, but I was very upset and actually she wanted to go off and play with her friends. Even though I wanted to hold her tight, I let her go. Leaving her to come back to the hospital was one of the hardest moments in weeks and I cried all the way back.

Friday, December 14th 2012
I am free! Joseph arrived to release me from my week with Andrew. Nice to see him albeit briefly, especially as he bought a mini bottle of red wine with him. Now I am off to the Globe Theatre for my Christmas work do. It felt very strange having to get ready in a hospital shower room with no hairdryer. I am mega-tired, but I am looking forward to going out, eating a delicious meal and talking to grown-

ups about something other than cancer. Most of all, I am looking forward to a weekend with Clara.

I saw a poster on a bus stop for Cancer Research's Dryathlon. I saw it and thought YES, I should do that; it should be easy, especially if we are in hospital again! However, if we are at home, it will be very hard. A glass of wine helps a lot at the end of a long day, but raising money to find a cure for cancer will help me more. If you would like to join in and be a dryathlete with me that would be delightful; if not, I would love you to "buy me a glass of wine" in a donation towards an important charity.

Sunday, December 16th 2012

An ambulance has been booked to take Andrew back to the Royal Marsden tomorrow for his next lot of vincristine chemo, which presumably means he can then come home - fingers crossed, please! I am looking forward to seeing my husband for more than ten minutes.

Clara and I had a lovely girl's weekend at Kelsey Park, eating in the French Cafe, slobbing about in pyjamas, watching Strictly Come Dancing, eating curry, partying with neighbours and popping to the shops. Most of all, a massive thank you to my brother and parents for doing much needed, hugely helpful DIY and odd jobs all weekend. I am looking forward to being joined by the boys tomorrow and seeing my husband.

My friend Cath has set up a Facebook page called 'Pints for Andrew', which is such a lovely idea!

The lovely Andrew is having a very rough time of it at the moment. He was diagnosed with leukaemia and, since then, he has been amazing, brave and strong and so have his parents. Andrew needs regular blood transfusions for the foreseeable future. This is where you can help. Can you be brave and strong like Andrew?

I'd like to get people to join this group and post whenever they donate blood. Andrew's parents will let us know when he has had a transfusion and I will keep a tally in order for us to keep up with Andrew. So, for every donation Andrew receives, I hope we can make a donation. Please post every time you donate, but also please add any donations you have made since 3rd October 2012. I appreciate not everyone is able to donate for various reasons; if you can't, could you please nominate someone to donate on your behalf; it could be a partner, relative, friend or even work-mate.

I'll kick it off. Andrew has had nine transfusions so far. I have given one donation. So we need eight more to keep up with him.

Monday, December 17th 2012
My little ray of sunshine is at the Royal Marsden and looking so much better. We are due back at the Queen Elizabeth in Woolwich tonight; everything is improving but not enough for us to be released yet. Home tomorrow?

Tuesday, December 18th 2012
Andrew is Home!

Wednesday, December 19th 2012

We had a visit from my neighbour, Clare, her sister, Emma, and some children carolling to raise funds for the Royal Marsden in Andrew's honour; they sang beautifully and were drenched from the rain; that is commitment for you.

Thursday, December 20th 2012

I am up with Clara who is being sick, so the Christmas holidays have come early and hopefully Andrew won't catch it.

Friday, December 21st 2012

A few weeks ago I nominated Andrew for a Cancer Research Star Award. Two packages arrived today. Andrew's contained a silver star shaped trophy, a T-shirt, a certificate with the signatures of various famous people at the bottom, and a £50 TK Maxx voucher. Clara also received a special certificate and a T-shirt. She was thrilled. They are both stars in my eyes.

Saturday, December 22nd 2012

We have had a lovely day, cooking mince pies and a half price Christmas cake kit from Waitrose. Andrew and I napped whilst Clara and Joseph swam; they almost had the pool to themselves. This was all followed by a fire whilst watching last week's Strictly Come Dancing with sherry and nibbles. I am grateful to be at home with my family; long may it last.

Sunday, December 23rd 2012

We have cooked a lot today - portions of chilli and chicken curry for the freezer, which we will use on our next surprise trip to hospital; lemon curd for gifts, and a Nigella ham in coke, as well as the three meals we have eaten. Andrew is walking around a lot more now; he is still wobbly but is even climbing a bit. He can now sit up on his own again. We have a lot of brilliant toys on loan from Cath. They kept us amused for a few hours. I realise I have not been out of the house since Wednesday. I am still grateful to be at home, especially as a few of the Royal Marsden families have been admitted in the last forty-eight hours – I am thinking of you all. We are off to the Royal Marsden tomorrow for another lot of vincristine chemo. Fingers crossed we can come home again quickly. I won't truly relax into Christmas until we do.

Monday, December 24th 2012

Andrew and I got home from the Royal Marsden only to be rung by the Queen Elizabeth in Woolwich to say we have to come in to redo the blood test. Andrew's platelet levels are low and he needs a transfusion. Hopefully the boys will be home by 8pm so we can have our Christmas Eve!

It is 22:40 and my boys are finally home! Merry Christmas everyone! May you get what you wished for and savour every moment you have with those you love.

Tuesday, December 25th 2012

We have had a fabulous Christmas day, mainly thanks to my parents who spoiled us all rotten. Thank you to Joseph who somehow managed to find the time to go shopping for presents. Both children are completely zonked out now. We will follow them shortly.

Wednesday, December 26th 2012

Here we go again. Andrew spiked a temperature of 38.8, so we are going back to the local hospital for a two-night stay whilst they grow blood cultures to find the source of infection.

Thursday, December 27th 2012

Joseph and I have swapped shifts, so I am at home with Clara. Andrew's temperature has stayed at about 37.4 for most the day, going neither up to the 'febrile' 38 degrees nor down to the normal 36 degrees which the doctors would like. So hopefully, if nothing horrid grows from the blood cultures, he will be home tomorrow. His high temperature on Boxing Day was probably a result of not drinking enough on Christmas day.

He is still neutropenic. His neutrophils are 0.0, so non-existent, which means he has no immune system whatsoever to fight infection. I was disappointed when he was taken back into hospital, as Joseph and I were finally going to have some time at home together, as a family, but it was not to be. The constant separation from Joseph and the dividing of the family is mentally exhausting. It seems never ending and I just want a break and to be normal again. We were press ganged into this cancer life and I want off the ship.

On Monday we start the next two weeks of horrid, horrid cytarabine, which last time caused Andrew to be taken in for two weeks, so I am sure this will be the beginning of another stint in the local hospital and our family will be split up again. Hopefully come February things might settle down. Please?

Friday, December 28th 2012

Today Clara and I made eight portions of turkey curry and eight portions of parsnip soup for the freezer, and six pints' worth of rice pudding. We bought Cancer Research cards and wrap for next year, bought and set two mouse traps, and delivered a present to the GP who originally started Andrew's diagnosis process. Joseph has been in hospital entertaining Andrew all day and is doing another night tonight; then they are coming home in the morning.

Saturday, December 29th 2012

One mouse evicted and two Berthoud boys home.

I understand now why people write in their Facebook status updates about doing a neutrophil dance. Andrew's are 0.0 and need to be 0.75 for the next stage of his chemotherapy: Consolidation Part Two. I am pleased next week isn't the week of horrors in terms of the chemotherapy mix, but I am worried we are delaying his recovery by another week. Then again, what is a week in relation to three years of chemotherapy?

Wednesday, January 2nd 2013

No news is good news. A lack of drugs means the old Andrew is returning slowly; it will all change next week when we start the next round of chemotherapy, but for now I am enjoying the downtime and happier days we are having together at home.

Thursday, January 3rd 2013

I was sick in the night so I am feeling very sorry for myself because I cannot be anywhere near Andrew. Throwing up and having a high temperature reminds me what it must be like for Andrew. I know I will recover in twenty-four hours, but he has felt like this on and off for three months now and will do so for the next three years. No wonder some days all he wants to do is sit on the sofa and watch TV.

Sunday, January 6th 2013
We had a lovely Berthoud Christmas weekend; Andrew and Clara were on tip-top form and enjoyed socialising. Andrew has been eating all weekend so I was a bit disappointed when we weighed him and he was 16.7kg – down from 20kg. The last time we weighed him, he was 17.9kg, so I thought he was going to be heavier not lighter. If he continues to lose weight, he will have to have an NG tube. I have started my Dryathlon. I am not drinking in January to raise money for Cancer Research UK. I wanted a drink yesterday with some yummy Stilton but I kept telling myself that I want a cure for cancer more. The community nurses are coming to take bloods at home tomorrow to tell us what Andrew's levels are like. I am expecting him to have to go and have a blood transfusion, so will probably miss my own blood donation sitting with him having his! If his neutrophils are high enough we can start Consolidation on Tuesday.

Monday, January 7th 2013
HB 10.7, WBC 3.6, platelets 395 and neutrophils 1.3. So no blood transfusion needed and we are all go to restart chemotherapy tomorrow with the next cycle. What a clever boy.

As I lay down on the couch to give a pint of blood for Andrew the lyrics "what have you done today to make you feel proud" from Proud by Heather Small came on. I choked back tears. I looked around the room at all the different people giving blood, wondering what motivated them to make an appointment and be there tonight. I am so grateful to everyone who donates. I always thought pints of blood were needed for people in A&E who had been in an accident, I had no idea there were children up and down the country needing blood transfusions on a daily basis.

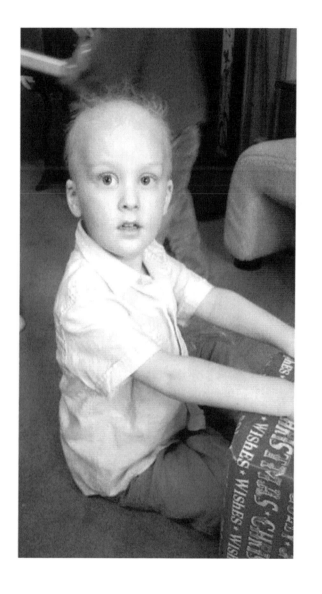

Chapter 5

Regimen C – Augmented Consolidation - Part 2

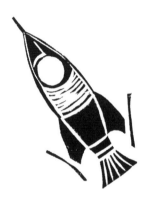

Skinny, bald and weak

Where did my 3-year-old go?

Precious, fragile boy

Tuesday, January 8th 2013

Home from the Royal Marsden - a 7.5-hour round trip. All went as well as it could, despite having to be in isolation again because of the C-Diff infection. Andrew has had two types of chemotherapy today: cyclophosphamide, which makes him feel sick, (hopefully reduced by the addition of ondansetron to trick his brain into feeling well), and cytarabine which causes the high temperatures. Fingers crossed he doesn't get a high temperature, which might mean we would have go to our local hospital for forty-eight hours. I hope he continues to eat and drink and he does not feel too nauseous. He will be given his third mercaptopurine chemo tonight an hour after he eats. The cytarabine has to be repeated at the same time (midday) on Wednesday, Thursday and Friday; then we start again next Tuesday.

Thursday, January 10th 2013

I don't want to jinx it, but suffice to say, we are all still at home. I worked from home today, answering emails and phone calls whilst entertaining Andrew.

Friday, January 11th 2013

I had a great day of respite away from the house and being a carer by going to work today. I am home now and Andrew is tucking into fish and chips, having had a lovely day with Daddy, Granny and Kesia. Joseph has taken Clara to a local roller disco in Orpington whilst we watch Ice Age 4. I am glad it is the weekend and hope it brings us more than 5 hours sleep a night.

Saturday, January 12th 2013

Another day at home. Andrew is walking more and more. Wearing shoes in the house gives him more stability, but he is still nervous about walking outside or venturing up or down a step. He is not napping much, which means he is less wakeful in the night, and neither Joseph nor I have slept in with him for the past few nights. It is fabulous to wake up next to my husband for a change. Andrew has been a STAR, taking his weekend medicine called co-trimoxazole (Septrin) today. (He must take three quarter tablets morning and night). We have been swallowing cut up paracetamol at the same time, to encourage him, and he tells us when to "ready, steady, go!" There were several points today where Clara and Andrew played together, like old times.

Sunday, January 13th 2013

I was pleased to hear today that Andrew has been accepted to receive four free tickets to Legoland thanks to the charity Merlin Magic Wand Awards for ill children (well done to me for applying on his behalf!): http://www.merlinsmagicwand.org/

Monday, January 14th 2013

We had a lovely play date with Andrew's chums this morning, the first since that day at the London Transport Museum over three months ago. He had bloods taken this morning and all were in the appropriate ranges. His HB is little low at 8.1, so he might need a transfusion next week; platelets are 164, but neutrophils are 1.9, which is an *increase* on last week so he has immunity still. What a clever boy he is! The last round of intensive chemotherapy starts tomorrow. The snowfall is exciting but I hope it doesn't hinder us getting to the Royal Marsden tomorrow or stop the community nurses from coming out on Wednesday, Thursday and Friday.

Tuesday, January 15th 2013
We are at the Royal Marsden again for cytarabine chemo today. Andrew has put on weight, only 0.35kg, but up not down - woohoo! That means we are not under threat of the NG tube. We were in and out in an hour!

Thursday, January 17th 2013
I worked this morning at one of the new academies around the corner from where we live. I thought Andrew looked pale when I picked him up at lunchtime from Mum's, so I asked the nurses to do an extra blood test and, in three days, everything has dropped. He is neutropenic again and will need a blood transfusion tomorrow. Luckily the nurse was able to take the extra blood needed for cross-matching, so Joseph and Andrew only have to go in once the blood has arrived. The transfusion will last four hours and will be pint number thirteen.

Friday, January 18th 2013
Andrew had the last of the sixteen doses of cytarabine chemo today - exhale - and no trips to the hospital with temperatures. He also had a four-hour blood transfusion and arrived home at 3pm. One hour later he was out playing in the snow with neighbours and joining in with the snowball fight. Aren't children utterly amazing?

We're at 15 pints for Andrew! Keep booking those appointments and doing your bit. For those that can't donate for a variety of reasons, please ask a family member, friend or work colleague to donate on your behalf; every donation counts and every donation saves a life.

Sunday, 20th January 2013

I cannot quite get my head around life being 'normal' at the moment. It certainly isn't the normal of four months ago, when there were no drugs to be taken every day, relentless sleepless nights and hospital trips. Yet it is a new normal, where blood transfusions are to be expected and our hospital bags are in the car, ready for a last minute trip. We still take every day as it comes and are grateful for small things, like all going to sleep at night under the same roof, singing songs at the kitchen table, Clara and Andrew sharing a bath together or days at the park with family.

The fact Andrew has cancer doesn't leave me; I find connections to it in everything I see, think and do. It has ramifications for the next three years and beyond. By the time we have finished this journey Andrew will have been ill for his whole lifetime over again. I wonder what normal will feel like in 2016.

Monday, 21st January 2013

It is not a good sign when the hospital phone with blood results less than three hours after the bloods are taken. Andrew's HB is 6.8, despite the transfusion on Friday, and his platelets are only 11, having been 384 last Monday. So tomorrow, at the Royal Marsden, he will have a blood transfusion, platelet transfusion, IV vincristine chemo and a PEG-asparaginase injection in his thigh. I think we will be there for some time.

Tuesday, 22nd January 2013

We are here at the Royal Marsden and have been since 9:30am. We have been seen by a doctor but have yet to start any transfusions and already it is approaching midday. At least we are not in isolation so are free to roam around and enjoy the playrooms.

Wednesday, 23rd January 2013 at 18:10

Yesterday I asked the doctor when Andrew was going to be allowed to go swimming again; she looked at me, amazed I had even asked the question. When Andrew was first diagnosed we were told 'normality' would resume after four months or so, which we had been thinking was February or March. We had expected he would be going back to preschool, swimming and going to sports clubs. However, we have since switched to the more intensive regimen.

Apparently now we should not expect 'normality' until we are in the Maintenance Stage. If there are no delays and everything goes as planned then Maintenance begins on 16th September 2013, which is when Andrew will be going to Balgowan Primary School. We will not be back at St James's Pre-School or Micro Sports or swimming, and we have seven more months of entertaining Andrew at home. Lucky or not for him, I am a primary school teacher so can at least teach him at home. What he won't be getting though are the formative years of social interactions with his peers.

Thursday, 24th January 2013

I left the house to go to work today in Peckham. Tomorrow I am back in Tottenham, meeting heads, observing some newly-qualified teachers and working with mentors. Andrew's blood transfusions have bumped him up to HB 8.6 and platelets 20: still low, but nothing now needs to be done until our next visit to the Royal Marsden on Tuesday.

Sunday, 27th January 2013

Clara and I are going to do the Cancer Research 'Race for Life' at Crystal Palace on Sunday 23rd June. If you would like to join Team Andrew let me know. We had a nice lunch at our local 'all you can eat' international buffet. Andrew's fortune cookie at the end read "life is a challenge - meet it". It certainly is and I think we are doing our best to do so.

Monday, 28th January 2013

Working two days a week gives me great flexibility. Now Joseph and I are doing all the childcare, and not using the child minder, I can work any two days or split my time across several days. I am working today in the school around the corner whilst Mum has Andrew for a few hours. Then I will be back home to collect him for his weekly blood test and to pick Clara up from school.

Andrew's blood results are back and a bag of platelets has been ordered for a transfusion tonight. We are booked in for 7:30pm. Luckily it is a quick one, taking only thirty minutes. It will be transfusion number sixteen.

At 20:59

Hurry up, platelets! They are coming from St George's in Tooting.

At 21:43

I feel like crying, as we still have no platelets, or rather they have arrived but are not enough – only the amount for a small baby, so we face another four-hour wait. I am just so utterly exhausted.

At 00:34

Oh, my word, Andrew had an allergic reaction to the platelets. The reaction started with him complaining of having itchy hands, which I thought nothing of. It was 11pm and I wanted him to go to sleep. He kept complaining, so I tried to get the night nurse, but she was busy with another patient. When I got back Andrew said his hands were hot, which they were, and that his head was itchy. In front of my eyes, his face, lips, eyes and hands were swelling until he resembled one of those Spitting Image puppets. He was flushed all over with a rash. I was petrified and he was crying. I was on my own, so pressed the emergency buzzer, unsure of what to do. No one came, so I had to console Andrew whilst also being desperate to get some help. I paced up and down; all of this was probably a matter of minutes, but it felt like hours and eventually I had to leave Andrew to get help. I stood outside the room where the nurse was accessing a new child. When she came out I burst into tears and said Andrew was having an allergic reaction. She swung into action and within minutes he was being given a Piriton and a steroid injection.

It was incredibly scary. I am now drinking hot, sweet tea whilst watching Dora the Explorer with Andrew and waiting for the Piriton and steroid to kick in. Today has probably been one of the worst days since diagnosis.

Tuesday, 29th January 2013

All the Berthouds are back at home. Our local hospital has rung to say we should come in tomorrow for a blood transfusion, two hours after the Royal Marsden said not to. So I said no! They consented to repeating bloods tomorrow and we will go from there. I will get the local nurses to come and do the bloods at home, and take some cross-match bloods too, so if a transfusion is needed I will only go in once his blood has actually arrived and is in the fridge.

Wednesday, 30th January 2013

HB is 7.2 today - teasing towards the transfusion cut off of 7.0, so a blood transfusion is being planned for tomorrow (Daddy's day at home) - pint number seventeen since diagnosis eighteen weeks ago.

Thursday, 31st January 2013

Thank you for all your donations towards my Dryathlon; I have raised £328.75 for Cancer Research.

Friday, 1st February 2013

My race for life pack arrived today. Clara doesn't seem best pleased with the idea, but I am sure once we are there, in sunny June, she will enjoy it? Thank you for the additional donations; I now have £375.39 for Cancer Research! Thank you to Cath for my box of delights which arrived this morning. Please send positive thoughts our way. We hope that Andrew will eat more today than he has over the last few days.

Saturday, 2nd February 2013

Cancer mummies: Andrew is off his food at the moment, so we are encouraging him to drink Scandishakes (high calorie, high energy drinks supplements). I know they are used to 'feed' children when they have an NG tube, which we do not have, but I wondered if anyone knew what amount of 'feed' a kid with an NG tube has in a day. I am wondering how much Andrew should drink in a day.

We were told that toddlers need a thousand calories per day, so we monitored how much my daughter ate and then topped up missing calories with the shakes via an NG tube.

My son has five hundred millilitres or seven hundred and fifty calories in a feed overnight, sometimes more. He hardly eats in the day. We are then meant to try and get another five hundred millilitres of fluid down his tube. Don't know if that helps. Good luck.

Sunday, 3rd February 2013

Joseph is off to Southampton to revel in the Super Bowl. The kids and I are on the sofa watching Annie and eating sweets.

I am cross with myself for only relating Andrew's mouth ulcer with his loss of appetite. For three days he has told me about the 'ouch' in his cheek and for three days he has not eaten. Today his lips are sore, so I have started swabbing his mouth with Corsodyl mouthwash, which he hates, but it gets the job done. Nothing to be done about the possible ulcers going all the way down his food pipe and into his tummy. My poor Andrew Bear.

Monday, 4ᵗʰ February 2013

There is lots of confusion at the Royal Marsden due to the week's break we had a while back. We were told last week that we were starting the next cycle, Escalating Capizzi, tomorrow, but actually it will be next week. So no lumbar puncture in the morning and a week of rest now. This is good, as it gives us a week to sort out the ulcers and Andrew's eating. We might still need to go in tomorrow, as we don't know if the appointment with our consultant has been rescheduled too. Andrew's HB has gone up and his platelets down, so he and Joseph have gone to have a platelet transfusion (the platelets have arrived and are in the fridge!).

Tuesday, 5ᵗʰ February 2013

I am taking Andrew to the local hospital to find out what is going on, as he is not a happy bunny today. The doctors seem unconcerned about Andrew; he does not have ulcers in his mouth, which is great, but does have something else which is making his mouth sore. They gave us Gelclair to use on it, which is like Bonjela. He perked up at the hospital BIG time, probably because there were new toys to play with and he had the total attention of both his parents. This shows that at home he is bored… as am I.

The doctors said we should feed Andrew whatever he wants rather than stick to the hospital shakes. I think we need to relax about his eating and not get stressed about it: easier said than done. He has eaten two yoghurts this afternoon. I have been to Waitrose and bought all sorts of full fat treats and snacks for him, so fingers crossed it will help. If you have any noisy plastic toys we could borrow for a while, to inject a bit of new fun into the playroom, I would be grateful, and I must book in some play dates. Andrew is neutropenic and probably will be for quite some time, but I think we need to see people. I certainly need some grown up company.

Thursday, 7th February 2013
I am holding my breath, as Andrew is eating a bowl of very soggy Weetabix; it is the first food he has fed himself voluntarily in a week.

Friday, 8th February 2013
When Andrew was lying on the floor screaming at bathtime, I saw a big white spot on the side of his swollen tongue - oral mucositis. It is no longer on the inside of his cheeks, so the new medicine is working.

Saturday, 9th February 2013
We had a delightful day at home: wine, cheese, cake, Eton mess, dancing, playing, moon sand, talking, sword fights, tea, fish and chips, running, chasing, hiding and most importantly, laughing. Thank you, Andy and Polly. You are great Godparents and friends. Just what we all needed.

Monday, 11th February 2013
Hi ho, hi ho it's off to our local we go - for another pint of platelets.

After waiting for two hours, I rang the community nurses at 11:30am to ask them when they were coming. They did not know they were supposed to come and take Andrew's bloods in readiness for a lumbar puncture tomorrow. They did then come and do them at 12:30pm. At 5pm I got a phone call from the local hospital saying Andrew's platelets were 37 and needed to be 50 for tomorrow's lumbar puncture. I needed to come in ASAP and have a cross-matching blood test done.

This nurse phoned the Royal Marsden to ask if the transfusion could be done there in the morning, but the doctor said no, so I arrived at 6:15pm.

The platelets were only ordered at 7:20pm. I was told no cross-match was needed, therefore the platelets could have been ordered at 5pm when nurse phoned me and I could have waited at home for them to arrive. I waited until 10:30pm for them to arrive, then waited until 11:30pm for the nurse to hook them up.

Why do I end up spending six hours in hospital for a thirty minute transfusion? So frustrating, but at least we are home now, even though it is 00:40. We need to be up at the Royal Marsden for an 8:15am lumbar puncture today.

Tuesday, 12ᵗʰ February 2013

We are at the Royal Marsden Hospital awaiting news of the next stage of Andrew's chemotherapy, and waiting for Andrew to have his general anaesthetic for a lumbar puncture.

We have just been told that Andrew's blood results are too low to begin the next stage of chemo. We should not be here. I am beyond fuming. His platelets needed to be 75 naturally and not due to a transfusion, and his neutrophils needed to be 0.75 or more (they are 0.2).

The Doctors could not understand how a transfusion was deemed a sensible idea last night, or how it was agreed by the doctor at the Royal Marsden who should have known better. Andrew was so tired, grumpy and hungry; he was beastly whilst I talked to the doctor. He ended up hitting me hard and I burst into tears. A kind nurse took him off to find something to eat.

When we eventually got home I got a phone call at 4:30pm from the Princess Royal University in Bromley, Kent, asking me why a consultant there has been given some blood results from 21st January to look at. I told her I had no idea and bloods from three weeks ago were irrelevant now.

Not a good day.

Wednesday, 13th February 2013

The positives from yesterday (after a good night's sleep) are

1. A 30 minute one-to-one with our consultant.
2. Andrew is still in remission - e.g. the cancerous cells have gone - we are now preventing a relapse.
3. I know the dates for hospital visits for the next eight weeks.
4. Andrew's weight is in the fiftieth percentile for all children, which is normal (so there is no need for an NG tube).
5. We have one week more to build up his weight.
6. Maintenance will be in June (not September).
7. The number of transfusions he has been having is normal.
8. Everything is very much working as it should be and everyone is very pleased.

There is no point staying angry for long, as it doesn't help anyone in the long run. I have to stay positive!

Thursday, 14th February 2013

I am spending Valentine's Day in Tottenham working with the newly-qualified teachers and their mentors whilst having a much needed break from being Mummy and the stresses of the last few days. I am now winging my way home to see my family. It is nice to have space, and the opportunity to miss them. I am looking forward to my M&S meal for two and a glass of red wine.

Friday, 15th February 2013

Since I got home from work Andrew has not stopped eating and is even now demanding fish and chips, but he is not even on steroids! Not that I am complaining; I would so much rather have a child constantly eating than not eating at all, like last week.

Saturday, 16th February 2013

Clara, Andrew and I are having breakfast whilst Joseph has a lie in. We are having mini croissants and large cups of hot chocolate (coffee for me), and we feel a bit like we are in France. Wonderful, as this is the closest we will get to going away for a while.

Whilst driving the car this morning I called someone an "idiot" in ear shot of Clara. She asked me what an idiot was, so I explained the situation and told her she should not ever use the word. She told me she knew the f word, but only ever said it in her head! She whispered to me, "Mummy do you know the f word, you know, 'for goodness sakes'?".

Sunday, 17ᵗʰ February 2013

Cancer mummies: I am going to try the magic cream on Andrew tomorrow, instead of the cold spray before he is accessed, but I not done it before! Can anyone tell me what to do, e.g. how much and for how long?

Put it on for an hour beforehand and cover it, either with clear sticky dressings or cling film. I use cling film for my daughter, as she hates the dressings. It just needs to be covered, otherwise it dries out and isn't as effective. Try EMLA cream as well, if you can get it, as you don't need to put it in the fridge and our local nurses prefer it to Ametop. Since you don't need to refrigerate it, you can carry one with you always. I used to have them everywhere!

The Ametop worked a treat. We had no screams and he enjoyed the novelty of being wrapped in cling film.

Andrew loves singing and loved singing at pre-school. When he was diagnosed in October they were learning harvest songs, so we are stuck singing harvest songs: "Conkers… I'm collecting conkers", "big red combine harvester", and "red leaves falling" ad infinitum. At least, with a whole year out of school, by the time he starts at Balgowan Primary School in September, they will be learning harvest songs all over again so it will feel normal to him.

Monday, 18ᵗʰ February 2013 at 08:41

It is half term and we are off to Coolings Nature Trail today to look for the signs of spring; the last time we were there, it was September 30ᵗʰ 2012, the day before Andrew fell ill.

In order to start the new block of chemotherapy tomorrow Andrew's bloods need to be 0.75 neutrophils and 75 platelets. Instead they are 0.6 and 73. So we will be retesting tomorrow for a possible start on Wednesday; otherwise it means another deferment to next week.

Tuesday, 19th February 2013

HB is 0.8 and platelets are 80 today, so we are going to start the next cycle with a general anaesthetic, lumbar puncture and IV methotextrate tomorrow. Fingers crossed the horrid side effects don't present too quickly or too badly. Andrew's HB blood level is 7.8 and needs to be 8, so a late night blood transfusion needs to be done tonight - always the way.

Wednesday, 20th February 2013

Andrew is fresh-faced after going straight from the Queen Elizabeth in Woolwich at 6am to the Royal Marsden for 8am. The nurses have written his name on the board as 'Spiderman' Berthoud, which he loves; he is wearing a Spiderman T-shirt.

However, at the final moment we have been sent away AGAIN as Andrew's platelets are below 75 this morning. We have been deferred until next Tuesday. Nothing surprises me anymore.

Thursday, 21st February 2013

My two bouncy children were in bed by 6:45pm and Joseph is still at work, so I am flopped on the sofa with a bowl of mussels, warm ciabatta with butter and a beer in hand, watching Murder in Paradise. I am ready to relax and enjoy this moment.

Saturday, 23rd February 2013
Poor Clara has tonsillitis. She was very pleased to be ill (like Andrew) until she tasted the penicillin prescribed.

Monday, 25th February 2013 at 11:27
Bloods have been taken by the community nurses - fingers crossed everyone!

The results are in: HB 11.3, platelets 101 but neutrophils still only 0.6, so I am waiting to hear if they will let us start or not.

Aargh! So the new plan (number five) is to repeat bloods on Thursday to see if the neutrophils have gone up; if they have, he will have his lumbar puncture and IV methotrexate on Friday. If not, we will withhold the Septrin, which can lower neutrophils, and then repeat on Monday. We edge closer to April 14th (Clara's birthday) and May 3rd (Andrew's birthday) but can still hopefully avoid nasty chemotherapy on or near those dates.

Thursday, 28th February 2013
At the recruitment fair last month I was able to talk to the head teachers about the primary newly-qualified teacher training being offered and how I would like to change it to one day of training a month. Everyone agreed with the idea and so today all the NQTs came to Head Office and met me for their professional development day. I think they enjoyed going to the shops in their lunch hour too.

Andrew's blood results are HB 11.0, platelets 130 and neutrophils 1.2, so we are (drum roll) going to start the next block of chemotherapy tomorrow - but don't hold your breath! They are saying that today, but as we know, everything changes in a heartbeat. The great news is that Andrew is not neutropenic after being so, more or less, since November. We have another nil by mouth and early start off at the Royal Marsden tomorrow.

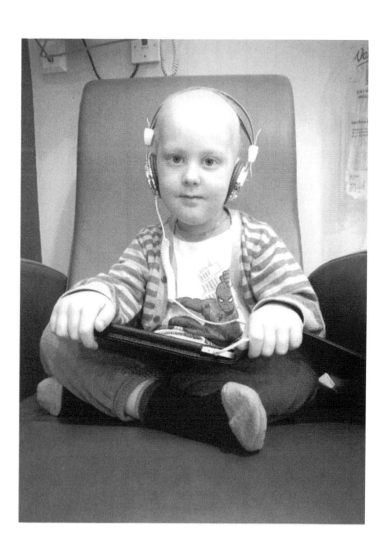

Chapter 6

Regimen C – Escalating Capizzi

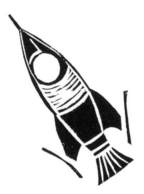

Flower gleam and glow

let the power shine on him,

Heal what has been hurt

Friday, 1ˢᵗ March 2013 at 13:56

We have arrived at the Royal Marsden and Andrew has been given the green light to have his lumbar puncture and Dose One of IV methotrexate – 100mg.

Whilst Andrew was munching his post-operation ham sandwich and Coco Pops, I noticed, on Andrew's new flow chart, that it says that end of treatment is three years from the start of Escalating Capizzi. So that means 20th February 2016. It is brilliant to have an end date, even though the date is nearly three years away and Andrew will be two months off being seven years old. At least I can start to mentally tick off the years, months, days and hours to the end.

Saturday, 2ⁿᵈ March, 2013

We have had a fantastic afternoon at Build-A-Bear and Zizzi in Bromley, all thanks to a charity called the Emily Ash Trust. This has been the first fun family event we have all enjoyed since diagnosis five months ago. The children love their bears: http://www.emilyashtrust.co.uk/

Sunday, 3ʳᵈ March 2013

Andrew was sick in the middle of the night but seems fine this morning, with no temperature. He has eaten a hearty breakfast. I am back in bed with the first coffee of the day after doing the early shift with the kids and allowing Joseph a lie in.

Monday, 4ᵗʰ March 2013

We were in and out of our local hospital this morning, in under an hour, for Andrew's vincristine chemo. We go to the Queen Elizabeth in Woolwich, which is part of a group of hospitals in administration. Every time we go, as a day patient, Andrew is given a choice of something from the 'present' box. Today he chose a big red car. The play team have no one fundraising for them and so love donations of any kind when they happen. There are seventy-five children, from Bromley, Greenwich and Bexley, on the 'books' who are treated on the oncology ward, I would like to gift some Easter eggs this year to those seventy-five children, so if anyone would like to buy an extra Easter egg and donate it to the ward I would be very grateful.

Wednesday, 6th March 2013

There is not much to report at the moment. Andrew is still at home, eating and scooting about. I am not sure all children at the beginning of Escalating Capizzi on Regimen C would be in the same state and it may all change at any minute. However, for now, all is well.

Sunday, 10th March 2013

Andrew's blood results are all healthy again. His HB is 10.8; his neutrophils are 2.4 (!) and platelets 89, so he will be having his second of five doses of horrid cytarabine chemo tomorrow.

Monday, 11th March 2013

We have had a fabulous morning. We went along to Songbirds Toddler Group at a local church for a play and a sing with my neighbour Clare and her son Dominic. The last time we were there was on the 1st October 2012, two days before Andrew was diagnosed. It was great to see him playing, eating them out of biscuits and singing his heart out. If it weren't for the bald head, you might not have known he was undergoing treatment for cancer.

At 15:48
We are at the Royal Marsden Hospital, waiting for a mix of chemotherapy treatments: Dose Two of IV methotrexate – 150mg today - and vincristine chemo. There is no TV, the IPad has run out of battery and Andrew has just thrown up all over the playroom toilet floor. Give me strength.

Wednesday, 13th March 2013
We had a bad last night. Andrew was awake for ages with a hurty tummy. He is not eating this morning and his tummy is still hurting. Poor Bear. Horrid cytarabine.

I have reached one hundred Easter eggs now. Amazing! Thanks to all who have contributed. The Queen Elizabeth in Woolwich are very grateful. I will take the surplus to the Royal Marsden when I go next week.

It is 9pm and we are on temperature watch - Andrew's is 37.9. At 38.5 he has to go to hospital; fingers crossed it doesn't creep up, please.

Friday, 15th March 2013
I worked in Chafford Hundred, Essex, again today, where I was moderating Year Six writing books. I have come home now to my clan who are all still well and bouncing about; we dodged a bullet there. Andrew's temperature was 37.2 this morning. Phew. It was a useful reminder for us all about how susceptible Andrew still is to infection and how even a cold could land us up in the Queen Elizabeth for forty-eight hours. I feel a celebratory glass of wine coming on whilst ordering some more hand sanitizer.

Sunday, 17ᵗʰ March 2013

My temperature is the same as Andrew's was on Thursday night. At least I can take some paracetamol (we are not allowed to give him any Calpol for the next three years unless prescribed by a doctor in hospital) and I am glad no one has to keep an eye on me or whisk me into hospital. I need an early night in my own bed and a hot drink.

Thank you to the children at a local Primary School who had a 'bring and buy' sale and raised £173.30 in half an hour! Their Eco Club are sending half of the money raised to Cancer Research UK on Andrew's behalf.

Tuesday, 19ᵗʰ March 2013

Andrew had an almighty tantrum from 8:45am until 9:15am on the way to school, causing Clara to cry. He seems to have one tantrum a day at the moment. The tantrums are exhausting for me, as a parent, but I understand they are Andrew's way of coping with everything which is happening to him; he is trying to regain control. Unfortunately, he is trying to control things that he has no control over, like Clara leaving and getting to school on time. I need to try and create situations where he can have a choice and a sense of control.

The nurses have been to take bloods, so now we are waiting to hear if Andrew's blood results mean he can have Dose Three of IV methotrexate on Thursday… He is currently tucking into his third bag of salt and vinegar crisps. He is definitely controlling his food.

Wednesday, 20th March 2013

It was Joseph's turn to take the children to school today. No tantrum today with daddy.

I had another great day with the newly-qualified teachers: what a great bunch of teachers they are. I am in my PJs now though, as I am ready to fall into bed and watch something mindless on BBC iPlayer.

Thursday, 21st March 2013

We are at the Royal Marsden today, to deliver the Easter eggs and for Andrew to have some less intense chemo - vincristine. He is missing Dose Three of IV methotrexate (200mg) because it is count dependent and his blood count is low already.

I am very proud of Andrew today for having a PEG-asparaginase injection in his leg with minimal fuss. Another boy screamed the room down! Andrew then walked all the way home from school. He recognised the words 'mum' and 'dad' and read them independently. I am also very proud of Clara after her parents evening; her teacher was again full of praise. A good day.

Friday, 22nd March 2013

After watching Tangled with the children, I have been thinking about how wonderful it would be if Rapunzel knocked on my front door and let Andrew hold her hair. He could sing the song which makes her hair glow and she could make him better. If only life was that magical or simple.

Saturday, 23rd March 2013

It has been a busy morning for Toy Monkey and Dr Andrew. Monkey has broken his wrist, so he had been given a Mr Wiggly and some sleepy medicine. Now he is ordering his post-operation food of bananas.

It makes me feel sad that Andrew's play involves things he should not know about as a three year old – but at least he has an outlet.

Sunday, 24th March 2013

In the absence of pre-school, I am busy devising a set of home school pre-school activities for Andrew and me to do over the next month or so; they are linked to spring, plants, growing, and the life-cycles of animals. I am excited – and hope he will be too! Tomorrow we shall be buying cress seeds, dried butter beans, daffodils and more moon sand.

Monday, 25th March 2013

I have celebrated Joseph's birthday on this day for the last twenty years, but tonight has been one of the best birthdays because we had two hours out for a delicious meal at Chapter One and we had a chance to chat. I was at home today with Andrew, benefitting from Joseph's new surround sound system. We had music playing in every room downstairs… hard life. I should have told Andrew the new sound system does not play 'The Wiggles' though.

Tuesday, 26th March 2013

Oh dear. We had such a nice morning at the Pre-School Easter Fair that Andrew was cross about coming home; he had a tantrum again (we've moved on from hitting me to biting me). Fortunately, it was short-lived and he was soon fast asleep, face down on the front door mat. He is now tucked up cosily, on the sofa, under his favourite blue blanket. I am sat on the sofa in an exhausted heap and really should be getting on with one of a hundred jobs on my to do list.

Wednesday, 27th March 2013
Andrew's bloods are all good today and his neutrophils are creeping up to 0.5. They need to be at 0.75 on Tuesday for the next lumbar puncture, so fingers crossed. If there was a correlation between the amount of chocolate consumed and neutrophils going up it would help.

Friday, 29th March 2013
I found my first grey hair this morning – I am somewhat amazed it has taken nearly six months since diagnosis to catch up with me. I hope I don't wake up in the morning white!

Sunday, 31st March 2013
I was up at 5:30am (6:30am, as the clocks have gone back an hour), watching Kung Fu Panda with Andrew, so I snuck back to bed for forty winks. However, I was followed by Clara who needed to know what was happening every day of the Easter holidays. We have created a Word document for her with a calendar of events. She is just like her mummy.

Monday, 1st April 2013
We took one quick trip to the Royal Marsden this morning for Andrew's bloods. The results are looking good, except for those neutrophils which are 0.69 and need to be 0.75

for him to have Dose Four of the IV methotrexate (250mg). Dose Five will hopefully be on April 12th.

Tuesday, 2nd April 2013

We are at the Royal Marsden Hospital, in the playroom with Andrew, who is nil by mouth and waiting for a lumbar puncture. The smell of burnt toast from the parent's kitchen is torture for him and me. We won't be having Dose Four of IV methotrexate either.

It is midday and Andrew is back from theatre and on a Coco Pops eating marathon. Gosh, I love him.

Wednesday, 3rd April 2013

We are back from a trip to our local hospital for vincristine chemo; this is our third day in a row of hospital visits.

Thursday, 4th April 2013

I wish we could go away and have a break, like most people are doing during the Easter holidays, but we plod on. Since Andrew had IV methotrexate on Tuesday, he has been in high spirits and there have been no tantrums. He has been sleeping at night, but he has also been sick, which seems to be part and parcel of the side effects. Despite the anti-sickness medicine, he is sick once a day for two days. We spent the afternoon putting together Clara's birthday party bags. It is very early in the month to be getting them ready, but the activity kept them both busy for an hour whilst the snow fell silently outside. I am looking forward to a mummy and daughter roller disco in Orpington tomorrow afternoon.

Saturday, 6th April 2013

Cancer Mummies: We are booked into the Legoland hotel for Andrew's birthday on May 3rd and will be going into the park on Saturday 4th. Has anyone been with their child yet? I am wondering whether to use the Q-Bot Ride Reservation Service, but then a friend told me to go to the front of the lines and tell them about Andrew having cancer and being neutropenic.

We have been to Legoland. All we did was take a letter from the consultant at the local hospital explaining my daughter shouldn't be out in the sun and couldn't stand or walk for any period of time. Go to Guest Services, which is on the right hand side as you go through the turnstiles, and they will issue your family with a wristband. You go to the exit of the rides and they let you straight on. Have a good time!

An adult carer gets in free so long as you take your diagnosis letter with you the first time you visit in a year – it is then stored for the remainder of the season.

Sunday, 7th April 2013

We are very excited to have won, in the bid, a set of tickets for Number One court at Wimbledon on the last Saturday of Tennis! That is a nice treat for Joseph and I to look forward to.

Tuesday, 9th April 2013

My friend Kate has kindly offered her garden for a charity event in Andrew's honour, to raise money for The Royal Marsden, in Sutton.

Please come to our garden party (entrance though the side-gate on Cedars Road).

£1 entrance per person (under 1s free)

Free bouncy castle for children

Stalls to include:

Pampered Chef, Usborne Books, Phoenix Cards, Jewellery and Neal's Yard Cosmetics

BBQ and Beer Tent

Homemade cake stalls and tea/coffee

Raffle

Wednesday, 10th April 2013

Andrew's weekly blood results are back and neutrophils are 0.2 and platelets 41, so there will be no Dose Five of IV methotrexate on Friday and we are back in home isolation again until his neutrophils are up. Luckily the Easter holidays are nearly over. I feel so sorry for Clara as she either has to be stuck at home with us or parcelled out with friends. It means that, of this phase, Escalating Capizzi, we have only managed the first two doses of methotrexate out of a possible five. Everyone says it doesn't matter, as they only give a patient what their body can tolerate, but I can't help feeling that more would have been merrier.

Friday, 12th April 2013

We are at the Royal Marsden Hospital so Andrew can have vincristine chemo and an echocardiogram of his heart. He had to have various sticky pads placed all over his chest and then be connected up to the computer. He lay very still for about an hour whilst the doctor took lots of readings. He is currently cheekily eating my tuna baguette, whilst waiting for his chemotherapy. I visited the Royal Marsden Charity fundraising room, so I am kitted out with the Royal

Marsden Charity banners, balloons, T-shirts and collection boxes for the garden party - woohoo!

Dan (Cath's husband) *gave platelets today: enough to give ten child platelet transfusions! He gave three donations, which he was told will be divided into ten children's donations, as his platelets are suitable for kids. Apparently some people have a residual virus in their blood which makes their platelets only suitable for adults. Interesting stuff!*

Saturday, 13th April 2013

I am very emotional about my baby girl turning six years old tomorrow. Where oh where has all that time gone? I am looking forward to a day of little girl treats, as she deserves to be spoilt rotten. She is an incredible sister and daughter. We have bought Clara a trampoline for her birthday, as we thought it would be a way of giving Andrew some exercise. When he is very cross, he can go and shout at the sky.

Monday, 15th April 2013

The children have been out on the birthday trampoline since 8am. We had lunch at Coolings Nature Trail, then rushed home to see the community nurses for some bloods. Andrew is having small nose bleeds and has a few bruises on his head, which suggest he needs platelets soon. His port bled for quite a while after the needle was removed too.

Thursday, 18th April 2013

It is not much of a surprise as he is a sibling, but it is still nice to know Andrew has a place at Balgowan Primary School for September.

Friday, 19th April 2013

What a difference from Monday! Andrew's bloods are all up: his HB is 7.5, so there is still no need for a pint of the red stuff; his platelets have risen from 54 to 135 and his neutrophils from 0.1 to 0.6. They will probably reach the 0.75 required for his next lumbar puncture on Thursday. This is all good news.

Sunday, 21st April 2013

We had a lovely, 'normal' weekend in our sunny garden. The children spent hours bouncing on the trampoline. We took Clara to the shops to spend her birthday money. I made a beef stew, roast chicken, lasagne and cakes; Andrew even ate his first vegetables in six months. I am glad Andrew is willing to wear a cap or else I would have had to cover his bald head in sun cream. Happy days.

Monday, 22nd April 2013

Andrew didn't want a nap today but he did want his pillow, blue blanket, two special teddies and the curtains closed. Needless to say, he is now fast asleep on the sofa.

Tuesday, 23rd April 2013

Andrew's neutrophils are low again, at 0.2, so the next stage of treatment, called Delayed Intensification, has been delayed (!) and we have no lumbar puncture or chemotherapy this week.

Wednesday, 24th April 2013

Andrew's lumbar puncture and chemotherapy have been rearranged for next week. Bloods will be taken on Monday; his lumbar puncture will be on Tuesday, his chemotherapy on Wednesday and then his fourth Birthday will be on

Friday! Joseph and I will be getting some work done in between.

Thursday, 25th April 2013

I am truly touched by the number of people who must think about Andrew and Team Berthoud on a daily basis: those of you still donating blood for him, liking photos I post on Facebook, coming to the garden party in May, sponsoring Clara for her Race for Life in June, seeing us at school, sending Andrew cards or just keeping me sane on Facebook. It is nice to know you are all still there for us in your own way, six months on, and it makes the hard moments or worries in the middle of the night so much easier.

Sunday, 28th April 2013

Joseph and I are gearing up for a very busy, exhausting and emotional week. Let's hope it involves more sleep than last week, else we shall be (even more of) a wreck by the end. Neither of us are regularly getting eight hours of good-quality sleep.

Monday, 29th April 2013

Andrew is wrapped up in cling film, waiting for the nurses to access his port and take some blood. The blood will then be taken to the Beckenham Beacon Hospital, where it is couriered to the Princess Royal University Hospital in Farnborough; they then process it and send the results to the Queen Elizabeth in Woolwich. I will get a phone call to tell me the results at about 3pm. Marvellous!

We are all go for the lumbar puncture tomorrow, and the beginning of the next stage, called Delayed Intensification – Andrew's Neutrophils are 0.9.

Monday, 29th April 2013

I am looking forward to an hour of peace, being able to sit down whilst reading a book and think my own thoughts with no one making any demands of me other than the nurses who will take my pint of blood. I am sitting in one of the new fancy recliners they have now for blood donors. I want to stand up and shout, "Thank you for giving blood. My son has cancer and it means such a lot that you are here!" Maybe I will next time.

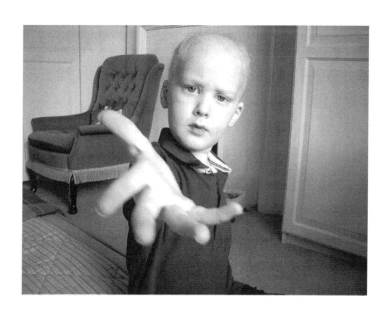

Chapter 7

Regimen C – Delayed Intensification

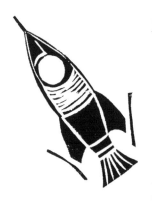

"Feed me, feed me" said

The hungry caterpillar

Munch munch munch munch munch!

Tuesday, 30th April 2013

The lumbar puncture and chemotherapy were successful at the Royal Marsden today. Andrew slept for three hours on the way home and has only woken up because I needed to go and pick up Clara from school. He has had his anti-sickness tablet to try and prevent him vomiting post-chemotherapy. He had a new chemotherapy today, called doxorubicin, which is red and makes his wee turn red for forty-eight hours or so - fun!

He was not given steroids today because the doctors have given us steroids in liquid form, instead of the tablets which Andrew prefers, so hopefully the Queen Elizabeth at Woolwich will give us the tablets tomorrow. Everyone is surprised a three-year-old takes tablets. We are so used to it now, but I must remember to tell each new nurse and doctor, otherwise they automatically give us the liquid steroids. We saw Andrew's consultant who said his cerebrospinal fluid (CSF) from the last lumbar puncture was still clear, which means there is still no sign of the cancer returning and he is still in remission.

Wednesday, 1st May 2013

We are at Queen Elizabeth Hospital after a 5am blue light ambulance trip with Andrew who woke up, in the middle of the night, coughing and in pain. Whilst we were on the phone to the Queen Elizabeth, Andrew flopped onto the bed, blue and struggling to breathe. Joseph hung up and dialled 999 immediately. The ambulance arrived within minutes.

Andrew has suspected croup, but hopefully we will be home later, as he has no temperature. Croup is treatable with a seven-day course of steroids, which we were due to start today anyway. It was tremendously scary and I am still running on adrenaline.

Thursday, 2nd May 2013
I had a great day at work in Penge and Peckham. I caught up on all my admin for the week this evening too. I hope tomorrow morning won't be the fourth 5am start of the week, but I think we will have one very excited birthday boy. You should see his pile of presents and cards!

Friday, 3rd May 2013
Happy Fourth Birthday, Andrew! Thank you for all the cards and presents, everyone. Andrew was so hyper when he saw them all. He is now fast asleep on the sofa. We are looking forward to picking up Clara from school later and continuing the birthday fun with a surprise weekend away.

Four very excited Berthouds have arrived at the Legoland hotel in Windsor. This is our first family night away since diagnosis on October 3rd 2012. I have nervous and excited butterflies in my tummy! Thank you Merlin Magic Wand for the tickets to the park: http://www.merlinsmagicwand. org/

Saturday, 4th May 2013
May the fourth be with you! I had no idea it was Star Wars weekend when we booked the hotel room. I am not sure who is more excited, us or the children! We were sitting, having our buffet breakfast, when I sensed some excitement behind me. I turned around and almost leapt out of my seat when three stormtroopers, Obi-Wan Kenobi and Darth Vader walked into the room. What a special day!

Joseph and a nervous Andrew queued up to meet them, and said, "Hello Darth Vader." He was quick to remind them his name was Lord Vader. They then walked up to Boba Fett, who was standing by the croissants, and asked him "what do bounty hunters eat for breakfast?" Boba Fett replied, "rebels."

Sunday, 5th May 2013

Cancer Mummies: Advice, please. Andrew is five days into Delayed Intensification, and is sleepy and down. We have been to Legoland and I know the dexamethasone can make him depressed but we've heard nothing about lethargy and tiredness. Is it the steroids or maybe the doxorubicin? I was expecting him to be running about, shouting, hitting, and eating loads.

The second and third week of DI, my son was knackered and really negative. He would put himself to bed at 4 pm. Try not to worry.

Steroids work in mysterious ways – they leave our son very emotional. Sometimes he is lost in his own world - lolling. Steroids, given late in the evening, play havoc with sleep patterns. They should not be given after 6pm. Dox used to leave him feeling sick.

Monday, 6th May 2013

Today has been a fabulous day for getting jobs done in the house and garden. A massive thanks to Mum and Dad for helping out. Andrew's steroids are making him feel very low, lethargic, tired, cold and a bit hungry. He needs to be held or cuddled all the time and must have eaten six scrambled eggs today. The last two doses are tomorrow and then we have a week's break. Andrew should spring back to his old self quite quickly. I told Clara she could have two pence for every dandelion she picked in the garden, not realising that she would find two hundred and nineteen! Andrew has more doxorubicin and vincristine chemo at the Royal Marsden tomorrow with Daddy, and I am off to interview newly-qualified teachers in Chafford Hundred. There is never a dull moment.

Saturday, 11ᵗʰ May 2013

I need sleep. Andrew always woke once a night before he had cancer. In the early days of the diagnosis, he slept badly and would often be awake for two hours in the night. However, seven months in, he still wakes frequently, making demands or needing a cuddle. I don't know whether it is part of the cancer treatment, at this stage, and whether to be sympathetic or get tough and do some sleep training.

Monday, 13ᵗʰ May 2013

We are off to our local hospital with Andrew who has a temperature of 38.6.

Andrews neutrophils are 0.0 so he has no immunity whatsoever; his platelets are 17 and his HB, 8.1. So a forty-eight hour stay at Hotel Woolwich is needed. I think it likely we will top up his platelets whilst we're here too, as they are low. Will we ever get a break to catch up on ourselves?

Andrew fell asleep at 6pm, so I managed an hour's sleep, between 6pm and 7pm, then another hour between 8:30pm and 9:30pm. There is no sign of his temperature returning at the moment. More IV antibiotics are needed at midnight. The main lights in the corridor have been turned off, so it is a lot darker now. It is 10pm so I will try and get two more hours sleep.

Tuesday, 14th May 2013 at 07:00

Morning. The 6am observations and IV antibiotics have been done. Andrew's temperature is still OK at 37.5 degrees. Andrew is on his second bowl of cereal with strawberries and raspberries. I had a six hour run of sleep between 12am and 6am, probably the most I have had in a row for a while. I am glad I fashioned blackout blinds out of blankets to stop the room getting light early.

At 10:53

Temperature is still 38.1 degrees.

At 23:04

One screaming child in the room next door, nurses who put the room's main light on and talk in normal, not whispered, voices, and a platelet transfusion to be done at 11pm. Fun. Not.

Wednesday, 15th May 2013

Sorry for going quiet - the data allowance on my phone was all used up because I was answering work emails; there is no Wi-Fi in the hospital. I am home now and Andrew is with Daddy. Andrew is in high spirits and eating. We have to wait forty-eight hours before we can come home though. Hopefully that will be tomorrow morning, although he might need a blood transfusion first. It has been a hard week, especially for Clara. I took her to school and then disappeared with Andrew for two days. She has had a new teacher this week too, so it is all change at home and at school.

Thursday, 16th May 2013

I picked Andrew up at midday and waited for the results of his chest X-ray (which should have been done when we arrived, not as we're leaving). They were clear with no sign of infection. The C-reactive protein (CRP) indicator of infection is low, at 14, and his cultures grew nothing, showing a negative result for infection. We have been prescribed inhalers, as his cough is probably linked to asthma. We waited and waited for discharge, so much so that in the end, I left to collect Clara from school.

On the way, Joseph texted to say Andrew's temperature was 38.3 and THEN it rose to 39.7! So he needs another forty-eight hours in hospital as per the protocol, even though he has no infection and it is only a viral cold. The doctors will increase his antibiotics to include an anti-fungal. Andrew is now due out on Sunday morning, but I have been told he can come out for the garden party if need be, as he has antibiotics at 12pm and 6pm. I am so frustrated because, if he didn't have cancer, I wouldn't even have taken him to the GP for a cold; I would be giving him Calpol at home. Now we all have to be separated for a week and he has to have lots of potentially unnecessary antibiotics for something viral.

Saturday, 18th May 2013

I am back home from another thirty-six-hour stint with Andrew. He spiked a temperature again, last night at 10pm, so we are in until Monday at least. The nurses thought it might be an infection in his line causing the problems, but then again maybe not. His antibiotics are being increased today; he is having about six different ones now. As a result, he is off his food and feeling pretty crummy. He is still coughing a lot, but the inhaler is making a small positive difference. I am grateful to everyone who is beavering away to get ready for the Royal Marsden garden party tomorrow. Andrew will hopefully be allowed out, but will have to go back to the Queen Elizabeth again afterwards.

Sunday, 19th May 2013

It was the Royal Marsden garden party today and Andrew was allowed to come! Weren't we lucky with the weather? What an incredible afternoon and turn out. Thanks to everyone for gazebos, cakes, donations and mostly for coming and spending your money and making the event such a huge success. We were so lucky with the generosity of those near and far. The total raised on the day is £2704.

Andrew had a brilliant afternoon and really didn't want to leave everyone, and then really really didn't want to go back to the hospital. To appease him I stopped off and bought him a cheese and tomato pizza to eat back in the room.

Monday, 20th May 2013

We have been discharged and are HOME!

Andrew has been missing pre-school and his formative years of play, so I am desperate for him to have activities to do in hospital that don't involve watching TV or playing on an Xbox. I started sifting through broken toys this week, throwing away the ones with no hope of repair, no batteries, or pieces missing, and then I rearranged the playroom into an early year's classroom environment for him. I am going to spend a bit of the money on buying some new toys for the oncology ward in Woolwich, but the rest will go to the Royal Marsden in Sutton.

Tuesday, 21st May 2013

I am the very proud owner of a new cloud-shaped charm for my Links of London bracelet. In the early days (and even now) we looked for all the positive moments, however tiny, and referred to them as being "silver linings on a big black cloud". I now have a permanent reminder to look for the positives in any situation.

Thursday, 23rd May 2013,

We are back at the Royal Marsden for more chemotherapy today. It seems never ending, as we have only just recovered from the last lot of intensive chemotherapy. More doxorubicin (red wee) today, vincristine and dexamethasone.

We are on Day One of high-dose steroids and Andrew is already very cuddly. Two weeks ago he was like this too, needing to be held, cuddled or carried all the time. It is much nicer than an Andrew who is angry and violent.

Friday, 24th May 2013

Andrew tolerated his chemotherapy on Tuesday without sickness. We have a well-timed break now, as it is half term, with no treatments scheduled until Tuesday 4th June. The school have made a date to get together and talk about his needs for September and we have been told who his teacher will be but are keeping it under our hats and have not told him.

Today is Day Three of high-dose steroids - with four days to go. Andrew is very sleepy and lethargic, a bit glum and irritable. He is not eating much but wants strange foods, like a Pizza Express pizza at 7am this morning. However today has been all about garlic butter and pesto straight from the jar.

Saturday, 25th May 2013

Today my hungry caterpillar ate two Pizza Express pizzas (yes, one at 7am again), five scrambled eggs, four dough balls, seven fish fingers, some chips, one cupcake and four mini plum tomatoes.

Andrew's eyes are troubling him; he blinks a lot and is very photo-sensitive. He needs sunglasses, even though it is not sunny, and the area under his eyes, where bags would be, is very red. He looks drugged up.

Monday, 27th May 2013
At 06:48

I was up at 5am with Andrew "Don't say it is not waking up time... I am not tired and I want to go downstairs" Berthoud. Then I was downstairs at 6am again, cooking sausages for him. The Very Hungry Caterpillar has eaten six sausages, six scotch pancakes with chocolate and strawberries, six dough balls, six scrambled eggs, one cake, half a large Pizza Express pizza and two bowls of honey Cheerios. It is not even dinner time! A hard-working mummy and an achy-legged boy.

Thank you to friends who ran ten kilometres, all for Andrew and CLIC Sargeant today.

Wednesday, 29th May 2013

The last week has been REALLY hard. I have been putting up with Andrew's constant hunger and depression, and he has lost the ability to walk again, so I am carrying him everywhere. He has long daytime naps and wakeful nights, early mornings and an appalling diet. Now though, it is harder because we have to train him out of all the bad habits:

1. Walk.
2. Eat vegetables and fruit to relieve your constipation
3. Eat meals with the rest of us, not what you fancy when you fancy it.
4. Eat at the table, not on a comfy chair because your back or legs hurt
5. Sleep on your own without the radio on
6. Play. Do not watch TV all the time
7. Give me some space and do not demand to be held or cuddled constantly

I hope it will all be fixed in a week or two, but I could do with a break. The up side to the steroids is that his neutrophils are 4.3, so we can at least go out and socialise.

Friday, 31st May 2013

Suddenly life is a little easier. Andrew is walking again. Phew! My back was beginning to spasm. He is going to the loo frequently and his tummy is still swollen, but that is probably all the PIZZA! He is sitting at the table with us to eat again. He is eating less, despite being egg, pizza and pancake obsessed. However, he now has the occasional sweet treat (a Marks and Spencer's chocolate ring doughnut) and even some fruit. We need to crack the sleep problem, but I am not holding my breath there. Joseph and I are off to the cinema tonight: a much needed escape.

Saturday, 1st June 2013
A book arrived in the post today called Wiggly's World. At a child's birthday party recently I got talking to another mum who, it turns out, works for a charity called Leukaemia and Lymphoma Research (now Bloodwise): https://bloodwise.org.uk/. She told me about the publication and said she would send me a copy. Clara and Andrew have both enjoyed reading the book with me, both shouting in excitement when it explains something Andrew has experienced, like an ECG, butterfly needle or numbing cream.

Monday, 3rd June 2013
Today we fell back down to earth with a bump. Andrew's neutrophils are 0.2, so he is neutropenic and unable to socialise again. His HB is 6.6, meaning he needs a blood transfusion in the morning. It is so important to grab nice days, like going to Legoland yesterday, when we can as we don't know what the next day will bring.

Wednesday, 5th June 2013
Andrew received some exciting post today. A signed photograph of Louis Smith! We all enjoyed watching Louis on Strictly Come Dancing so I wrote to his agent asking for a signed photograph to arrive for his birthday – it came today. Better late than never and Andrew is thrilled!

Thursday, 6th June 2013

It is all go at work at the moment. This year's newly-qualified teachers are about to complete their induction year, so they all need to be observed and signed off. Then we are recruiting and interviewing next year's, so I am planning recruitment and induction events, and next year's training programme. Granny, Grandad and Kesia have come to visit and help out with childcare. Andrew collected Clara dressed as his favourite X-men character, Wolverine, and got a lot of admiring glances and comments.

Sunday, 9th June 2013

Andrew has managed six nights in a row without waking up in the middle of the night for the first time EVER! Then this morning he got out of bed to go for a wee all by himself; he is growing up.

Monday, 10th June 2013

We had a meeting at Balgowan Primary School this morning with Andrew's teacher, teaching assistant, and community nurse to discuss his needs for September. The leaflet for parents and the medical plan I wrote and printed out were well received and covered all the main points clearly. His reception teacher is going to send all the washable construction home with staff to be run through dishwashers and will have the classroom deep cleaned.

This is Andrew. He is starting at Balgowan Primary School this September and will be in Mrs. Palmer's Class in Reception.

Andrew has leukaemia and will be in treatment until February 2016.

PLEASE READ THE FOLLOWING INFORMATION

Andrew is at risk from ALL infections, in particular chickenpox, shingles and measles. If your child has a known infection, but is well enough to attend school, please inform the school so Andrew can be kept at home. Andrew has something called a "port" near his left armpit. This is used to take blood and give medication. It is very sensitive to touch and can be uncomfortable after treatment.

Andrew has to take lots of medicines and some of them can affect his moods and behaviour. This can make him tired, emotional, angry or hungry: any one of these or all of them together and his reaction is different each time he takes the medicine.
Your child may notice that Andrew frequently leaves the classroom. This will be because of his health needs.

Please encourage your child to have good hygiene and hand washing skills. This will help to keep Andrew safe and well.

If you have any questions about Andrew or his illness, please feel free to contact me through the school.

Thank you,

Melody (Andrew's Mum)
Tuesday, 11ᵗʰ June 2013
We are off to the Royal Marsden tomorrow as Andrew's
blood test this morning gives us the green light. We are

The healthcare plan for staff:

Name : Andrew	D.O.B	Date written:	Review : ongoing
Need	Frequency	Action required	Action by
Medication Whilst at home Andrew takes the following medicines: Mercaptopurine – daily oral chemotherapy Methotrexate – monthly oral chemotherapy Septrin – weekly antibiotic Dexamethasone – monthly steroid Vincristine – chemotherapy injection into Mr wiggly monthly	No medication should be required at school. Andrew is not allowed Calpol or nurofen. Steroids can affect mood and behaviour whilst taking them, sometimes causing emotional changes and challenging behaviour (possible rage and depression) Vincristine can cause his legs to ache and make him feel nauseous.	Staff to be aware that Andrew is taking steroids Staff to be made aware if Andrew is experiencing any side effects from current medications	Parents to keep school informed of any side effects / behaviour changes Class staff to keep Andrew's parents informed of his progress in class

Need	Frequency	Action required	Action by
Absence	Weekly at home	Parents to make school aware of results of weekly blood test – neutropenia (0.5) or below he cannot come to school, low platelets mean he will bruise more easily and low HB means that he will be more tired and lethargic because he will be short of breath.	Parents
Blood tests			Parents School Office
		Parents to provide copy of regimen and known dates of absence for hospital appointments where known.	
Controlling contact with infection Andrew must not be exposed to infections such as chickenpox, shingles or measles Exposure to minor coughs and colds are inevitable and usually carry low risk to Andrew.	Drugs used to treat leukaemia interfere with the body's ability to cope with these infections	School to send parent letter to whole school advising of risk of bringing such infections in to school All staff must be made aware of the potential risks to Andrew to prevent exposure On notification of infection from another parent the school must inform Andrew's parents immediately Encourage good hand hygiene prior to meals and following use of bathroom. Allow Andrew to use the disabled toilet.	Headteacher CNs School administration staff / class teacher Parents to provide hand sanitisers.

Need	Frequency	Action required	Action by
Snacks As part of his treatment Andrew must take steroids. This increases his appetite and he requires regular snacks to satisfy his hunger. Mum will provide snacks for Andrew whilst at school	Andrew is given steroids by mouth for 5 days every month. These will be given by Andrew's parents at home. His hunger should settle after each course stops	When Andrew is hungry he should be allowed a snack Staff should be aware of communication from Andrew's parents that he is taking steroids	Reception class staff Andrew's parents must inform school that he is on steroids and provide snacks whilst at school
Controlling contact with infection Andrew is at risk of infection and needs immediate assistance if he feels unwell or hot.	Continuous risk whilst on treatment until March 2016.	Inform Andrew's teacher immediately if he complains of feeling unwell If thermometer available Take Andrew's temperature using digital thermometer and contact parent immediately If temp >38.0 or Andrew looks unwell and a parent is out of contact call local ward on xxx and notify ward staff. Transport to hospital immediately using ambulance if necessary. Inform crew that this child is known to Tiger Ward who are expecting him. Continue to contact parent.	Class staff Member of school staff to contact parent Parent to ensure contact from school is possible at all times barring unforeseen circumstances Parent to discuss Andrew's potential signs of illness and not only through high temperature Parents to give school a copy of ambulance letter for the ambulance crew.

Need	Frequency	Action required	Action by
Tiredness Andrew may tire easily and may require extra rest	Ongoing through treatment and for a while once treatment ends	Andrew will require somewhere quiet to rest for short periods Staff need to be aware of Andrew's need	Class staff
Need	Frequency	Action required	Action by
Potential damage to portacath (bubble) sited under the skin covering Andrew's chest	Ongoing whilst portacath (bubble) is in place	PE and playtime activity is safe whilst needle is not in however any bump to the area may need inspection and attention. If needle is in place Andrew will not attend school.	School staff to inform parent at time of any incident immediately Andrew's parent to inform and advise the school

Contact phone numbers

entering the last four weeks of intensive chemotherapy, so I am pleased, even though it is not going to be remotely nice for Andrew.

I take with me the £2704 raised from the garden party, I am keeping £300 back for the Tiger Ward playroom. Yes, our total raised was £3004. WOW.

When someone is generous with themselves towards us it makes us feel special and cared about. When someone can be generous in spite of what they are coping with themselves it inspires us to want to be more generous with ourselves and pass on the love. Thanks Melody for passing on the love.

This is the first time somebody has told me I am inspiring. I didn't set out to be inspiring. I am coping with an intensely stressful situation the only way I can. Joseph likes to tell people a story of life before we were married, when we decided, one weekend, to paint the small bathroom in our two-up two-down house in Bromley North. He imagined that we would spend the weekend in Homebase choosing paint colours; however, by Friday night, we had been to the shop, purchased the paint and put the first coat of white on the ceiling. We call this 'being a Head,' after my side of the family, (the Heads) who have a tendency to 'Just do it' rather than deliberate about it. It does mean I have a tendency to rush into things without thinking about the pros and cons.

As a teacher I liked to have a routine and follow my timetable. As a stay at home mum I craved routine and liked to know what I was doing the next day, week and month. One of the first purchases I made when Andrew was diagnosed was a new calendar. I threw away our pre-planned old life and set about planning for a new one. I wrote all the appointments down, then invested in some Tipp-ex to white out events, and eventually learnt to write in pencil, as appointments constantly changed.

When Andrew was diagnosed, I told people of his situation through texts, cancelling up and coming events in my diary.

"Cath, I won't be able to come out for dinner because Andrew has been diagnosed with leukaemia".

I have always been an organised person and I coped with the stress of diagnosis by going into hyper-organised mode. It gave me a focus, a distraction and it felt good to be doing something useful for the family in the middle of the crisis. Having an idea for raising money is easy; getting people to buy in to the fundraising and give money is harder. Luckily I have friends and family who are wonderfully supportive.

Wednesday, 12th June 2013
We are at the Royal Marsden for a lumbar puncture, cyclophosphamide and cytarabine chemotherapy, and high-dose steroids. It feels as if we are throwing everything at Andrew's cancer today – bring it on!

Thursday, 13th June 2013

Mr Wiggly goes into a portacath under Andrew's skin, which in turn sends the medicine directly into his heart and blood stream. This is how blood comes out too. Mr Wiggly doesn't normally stay in, but this week we have needed it for more cytarabine chemotherapy on Wednesday, Thursday, Friday, and Saturday and will need it Monday, Tuesday, Wednesday and Thursday next week!

Friday, 14th June 2013

I am fed up at missing out on the big Telford family camp this weekend and am saddened by the thought of not seeing Clara for two and a half days. Of course there is no way Andrew can go and Clara must be allowed to go and have fun with her cousins.

Andrew had his IV vincristine chemo at lunchtime and four more tablets of mercaptopurine chemo at bedtime. I had a great afternoon at work catching up with everyone whilst Andrew played with Mum and Dad at the park and in the garden (surprising after chemotherapy). Then I had some of my favourite wine and a dinner cooked by someone else - so one mile away from my house, I feel like I am on my own mini holiday.

Saturday, 15th June 2013

The last cytarabine chemo of the week was injected by the lovely Nurse at the Queen Elizabeth in Woolwich. I am so grateful that she came in on her day off to do this for us.

Sunday, 16th June 2013

Ross Hutchins has raised £130k so far today for The Royal Marsden through the 'Rally for Cancer' event and Team

Andrew has raised £1300 so far for Cancer Research's Race for Life next Sunday! Wow! Again I am moved by everyone's generosity, all for my little boy.

Monday, 17th June 2013

Despite a mixture of eleven types of chemotherapy in the last five days, Andrew's bloods are the best they have been for a while. HB 9.3, neutrophils 1.0 (so we can socialise) and platelets 95. Clever boy.

Tuesday, 18th June 2013

I am back again at the Royal Marsden Hospital with Andrew, who is due to have a lumbar puncture under general anaesthetic. Methotrexate chemo will be injected into his spine and another lot of vincristine chemo will be administered through Mr Wiggly. Every time we come I have to sign a declaration form to say that I agree to the procedure. Most of the time the doctor doesn't list off the known side effects of the treatment, but today she did. I know that Andrew could suffer headaches, back pain, fever, topical swelling and even paralysis as a result of the chemotherapy being injected into his spinal fluid, but I cannot refuse the life-saving treatment.

I am fed up of everyone staring at Andrew's bald head; we are three weeks off Maintenance - how long is it before his hair will come back? Andrew doesn't notice, but when random children come up and rub his head or point and say "you've got no hair", laugh and call him bald, it makes me MAD. Andrew has a birth mark on his head which we knew nothing about until he was completely shiny bald and I am glad to know about it.

Wednesday, 19th June 2013

Andrew scooted to school today, then we played in the local park. He had a play date with a friend and a photo session in the garden. A mum in Clara's class is doing a photography course and needed children for her case study. I offered Andrew and was thrilled she chose him. It will be superb to capture him right now, bald head and all. I had a chat with my friend Cath whilst the mum snapped away and now Andrew is bicycling to school. If it weren't for the chemotherapy at lunchtime it would almost be like I had woken up from a bad dream.

Friday, 21st June 2013

Woohoo! The last cytarabine and the last of the intensive chemotherapies have been injected. Now we have two years and nine months of the same maintenance drugs to prevent relapse.

Sunday, 23rd June 2013

I am so uplifted and emotional after Clara and I completed the 5km Race for Life at Crystal Palace in fifty-three minutes. She was INCREDIBLE! Thanks to everyone who came and joined in for Team Andrew. Thank you to all the children who finished, to the supporters who cheered us along, the families walking, and most of all Joseph and Andrew who kept appearing to spur us on. £2317 raised so far. WOW!

Tuesday, 25th June 2013

Today was Andrew's first taste of primary school. He went into his classroom and met his teacher. I was very apprehensive, meeting the other new parents, as Andrew is still completely bald, and I wondered what they must be thinking. Have they noticed his bald head? Do they realise it is because he has cancer? After a morning at school we then had an afternoon at the Royal Marsden for a blood and platelet transfusion; what an awesome little boy! However now Andrew is awake and in pain after this afternoon's vincristine chemo. Hopefully a codeine and a daddy sleeping on the truckle will make things better.

Wednesday, 26th June 2013
Andrew is having another pint of blood at the Queen Elizabeth Hospital. The blood had to be slowed down as the rate of resistance is too high. It should be minus something and it is nearly one hundred! Not a problem, but it is taking a long time. Blood can only be out of the fridge for four hours so that means we might not have enough blood in the time allowed.

Sixty-fourth pint donated by Debbie's husband - thanks! Andrew received a pint today so we're at 64-22.

This was Andrew's 22nd and final transfusion.

Monday, 1st July 2013
A year ago we were recovering from a magical night, celebrating our tenth wedding anniversary. Mum and Dad had a marquee in their garden – reminiscent of our wedding reception - to celebrate the establishment of Dad's new trust. The next day we invited all our family and friends to come and celebrate ten years of married life with us. Our friends played music whilst we danced a Ceilidh. It was the first time the children, only three and five years old at the time, had stayed up until nearly midnight. Everyone brought a dish or a pudding and we shared the meal. The children played in the garden whilst the grownups danced

into the night. It was a magical evening. Who knew, a year on, one of us would have completed nine months of gruelling chemotherapy? I wouldn't have believed it if you'd told me and I certainly would not have believed it to have been Andrew.

Tuesday, 2nd July 2013

A day at work for me and Joseph's turn to be a house husband. Andrew was at the Queen Elizabeth in Woolwich today for vincristine chemo in his port and to have bloods taken. His platelets are at a good level, but his neutrophils have dropped to 0.1.

Thursday, 4th July 2013

Over the past three days I have visited five schools, observed twelve newly-qualified teachers, examined twelve portfolios and given twelve lots of feedback. I am now on my way home to my three lovely Berthouds to see how much hair Andrew has grown in three days.

Friday, 5th July 2013

I am very proud of Clara who has a glowing end of year school report and has made 'exceptional effort and progress this year'. We are thrilled the school have been such a constant source of stability and inspiration to her throughout her year as a cancer sibling.

Monday, 8th July 2013

Andrew's blood results show everything is dropping or has dropped. His neutrophil levels are 0.0 so he has no immunity to infection at all. That and this heat mean a two-day stay at the Queen Elizabeth in Woolwich could be on the cards so he needs lots of rest, fluids and extra precautions to be taken. We were due at the Royal Marsden tomorrow, for the official beginning of Maintenance, but it has been delayed. Hopefully, in a week, everything will have picked up a bit, but it is a long climb to the 0.75 neutrophils needed for Maintenance to begin.

Tuesday, 9th July 2013

Andrew had a temperature of 39.4 at 2am so Joseph took him to Queen Elizabeth. We always stay for forty-eight hours after a high temperature, for blood cultures to grow (or not) and show the source of infection.

Wednesday, 10th July 2013

Andrew has not had a high temperature since we got here. He has forgotten what hungry feels like and instead thinks he is going to be sick. A handful of dry Cheerios soon sorts that out. We both slept deeply despite the two-hourly medical interruptions. Hopefully we will be allowed out for Clara's sports day this afternoon and maybe home in the morning if his temperature stays down. A morning of playroom tidying and rearranging for us! There is a play team at the Queen Elizabeth, but they are very busy with the main ward and the outpatients' departments which get more foot fall. The oncology play room doesn't always get tidied up so I like to have a sort through whenever we are in. I look for missing pieces to jigsaws, dice for games or DVDs for boxes. I throw out anything that is broken or missing too many pieces. I love sorting and rearranging and it gives me something to do.

Thursday, 11th July 2013

We are back home!

Thursday, 18th July 2013

Joseph and I enjoyed a hilarious night with Jason Manford in Tunbridge Wells. It felt great to laugh until it hurt. Andrew knew we were going out to see someone who would tell us jokes and wanted me to remember one of the jokes. I couldn't think of any at the end of the night to relay to him in the morning so instead sent Jason a message on Facebook and asked him for his favourite children's joke. His reply was:

What bees make milk? Boobies!

Friday, 19th July 2013

It has been a hard week for my state of mind. Andrew cannot go outside into the direct sun or get too hot (our hospital stint was due to him overheating, they think) and we cannot socialise because of his low immune system, so we are going to be stuck indoors, in the dark, attempting to keep the house cool, for most of the week. I had a bit of a panic about it on Wednesday and had to get out of the house. I ordered a new gazebo to give shade in the garden. It arrived today and has made a big difference. I have put it over the new paddling pool so Andrew can have the fun of the pool in the shade and keep cool. It is only three more school days until Andrew has Clara as his playmate for the summer. He misses having children to play with. His bloods will be retested on Monday. Fingers crossed the levels rise.

Saturday, 20th July 2013

Andrew is hungry today, which makes me think his blood counts are recovering. He is probably gearing up for the beginning of Maintenance, which starts with five days of steroids.

Sunday, 21st July 2013

Thank you Ben and Kay for organising a private screening of Despicable Me Two at the VUE in Croydon. It was very funny. How wonderful to be able to go to the cinema without worrying about strangers who might be infectious. There were so few of us that we had whole sections of the seating to ourselves. Joseph and I laughed a lot too. Laughter is the best medicine to relieve to stress.

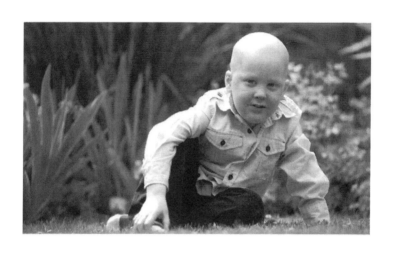

Chapter 8

Long Term Maintenance - Cycle 1

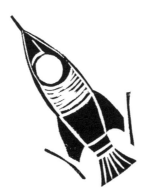

One child in this town

But ten mums on this playground

Cancer's everywhere

Tuesday, 23rd July 2013

We have made it to Long Term Maintenance! Andrew was diagnosed nine months and twenty days ago. Andrew will be having oral mercaptopurine chemo everyday now, at bedtime, an hour after his last food. Every three months we will go to the Royal Marsden at the beginning of a twelve-week cycle to be injected with vincristine chemo along with taking oral dexamethasone steroids for five days. We will then visit the Queen Elizabeth in Woolwich for the following two months to have the same vincristine and dex. Every three months we will visit to the Royal Marsden for a lumbar puncture for intrathecal methotrexate. We have twelve of these cycles and our end date is 20th February 2016.

Chemotherapy attacks rapidly growing cells to kill the cancer cells. However, it attacks all other rapidly growing cells in your body, like your hair, and the inside of your mouth and stomach. Hence the hair loss and ulcers in Andrew's mouth and stomach, causing weight loss. At diagnosis, Andrew weighed nineteen kilograms and, at his lowest point during intensive treatment, he weighed sixteen kilograms. The daily chemotherapy on Maintenance is not the same type that causes hair loss and ulcers. His hair has already begun to grow back. I wonder if it will be blonde and curly again or brown and straight, like mine.

Thursday, 25th July 2013

Andrew has white stripes across his fingernails. They are called leukonychia striata, a whitening of the nails in bands which run parallel to the nail base. The condition or damage is caused by chemotherapy and a very real sign that the intensive chemotherapy is leaving Andrew's body. Lots of cancer children have the white stripes often on their nails but sometimes in their hair too.

Sunday, 28th July 2013

I love dexamethasone week: Andrew's neutrophils are 6. No, not 0.6 - 6!

Tuesday, 30th July 2013

It is 7am and we were all up and off to the Royal Marsden for Andrew's general anaesthetic lumbar puncture and IV vincristine chemo. We don't need to be back here until October 15th 2013, by which time Andrew will have completed a month of school. The consultant told us we should now treat Andrew like a 'normal' boy, who should be socialising with his friends, swimming and going to school.

He also said Andrew will not be neutropenic so often, as the neutropenia will be controlled with daily medicine. Chicken pox, measles, shingles and infections which originate from his own body are still a big danger, but not coughs or colds from others. Our consultant suggested avoiding crowded places. The change of mindset back to 'normal' will be almost as hard adjusting to 'cancer,' in the beginning, but at least it will be more fun! We must still go to hospital if his temperature reaches 38.5, but will only stay in for forty-eight hours if he is neutropenic, as we can now give him oral antibiotics at home.

Friday, 1st August 2013

I am playing I Spy in the kitchen with the children.
Me: "I spy something beginning with W."

After a few guesses, Clara says, "Give me a clue."

Me: "They are on the inside and outside, and I can see fifteen of them."

Clara: "Wine!"

Saturday, 3rd August 2013

We have been for our first family swim in nine months. As luck would have it, Andrew's swim teacher was there and took him off for a ten-minute lesson, which she has offered to repeat. Andrew scooted to the pool with his swimmers in a rucksack on his back.

Sunday, 4th August 2013

We are at the Queen Elizabeth in Woolwich, having Andrew's weekly bloods done now, so as not to waste a moment tomorrow when I am with Amanda and Cath. Andrew's blood results show his neutrophils are 0.1, so we have to be careful about infection risks, especially as a holiday is looming. Andrew has no daily or weekly chemo until Monday, when he has his next blood test, and we can see if the counts have risen.

Friday, 16th August 2013

We are on the way home from a brilliant week in Battle, Hastings. We stayed in the Emily Ash Trust's caravan at Crowhurst Park. The Emily Ash Trust gives sick children normality during difficult times. A huge thanks to you for a much-needed break. We swam every day in the lovely indoor pool and the children tried water zorbing, which they loved. We visited Battle Abbey where we learnt to sword fight and visited the seafront to play on the penny slots. We ate breakfast and dinner on the sunny terrace outside of the caravan. Joseph and I both feel much more relaxed.

Saturday, 17th August 2013

Today is a momentous day. We are driving to the grandparents, in St. Osyth, for the first time since diagnosis. We are having a mini Berthoud camp in the garden, with cousins, to make up for Andrew missing out on the big family Telford Camp in July.

Tuesday, 20th August 2013

We are back at home and back at the Queen Elizabeth for another cycle of vincristine chemo and dex steroids.

Wednesday, 21st August 2013

Your Hero Made Super Picture # 12 is for Andrew who is currently battling acute lymphoblastic leukaemia (ALL) with the help of his big sister, Clara: http://www.yourheromadesuper.com/

I applied, a while ago, for Andrew and Clara to be turned into a super hero characters for a comic picture. Danny Warren's daughter, Naomi, was diagnosed with T cell acute lymphoblastic leukaemia (ALL) in February 2012, aged two, and ever since he has been paying it forward by creating stunning pictures. I received the picture he drew of Clara and Andrew via email during the interval of a performance at Sadler's Wells and a woman asked me why I was crying. I had to explain to her they were happy tears, as I was over the moon. I am going to get the image put onto canvas and hung in the playroom.

Thursday, 22nd August 2013

Andrew amazes me every day. We are halfway through steroid week and, so far, he has taken thirty tablets. No fuss. Yesterday he took nine of them all in one go.

Saturday, 24th August 2013

Steroid week is a double-edged sword. I know his neutrophils will be boosted, which means we can go out, yet he is very tired, cuddly, grumpy and unable to walk much more than a few metres again. When we are at home all he wants to do is watch TV or play on the Wii. This time around he has wanted to eat lots of beans on toast - but one tin is enough in a day.

Today we enjoyed the kids' cinema screening in the morning (even though Andrew choked on his popcorn and threw it all back up into the popcorn carton). I have recently found out about the Cinema Exhibitors Association or CEA card. I had to pay £10 for the card, which lasts a year but it gives me one free adult ticket when I take Andrew to the cinema: https://ceacard.co.uk/

This afternoon we swam at the local Family Splash session. The buoyancy of the water in the pool seems to ease Andrew's leg pain. Luckily he naps during dexamethasone week too, which gives us all a break from caring for his needs. The last tablet is due tomorrow morning. Next month's dex is being brought forward a week, as he is due to have it in the same week as starting school. Bringing it forward means he has four weeks to settle in before the October steroid side effects take hold.

Monday, 26th August 2013

Twenty-four hours post-steroids my little boy is back, bouncing, and being so grown up. We are off to meet cousins for the day at Stansted Mountfitchet castle.

Thursday, 29th August 2013

I noticed today how hairy Andrew's legs are. I have been so obsessed with his head hair loss and regrowth that I had not noticed. His face is covered in fine hairs now and his eyebrows are thicker and growing out in all directions. I understand now why his consultant at the Queen Elizabeth told me about asking the boys to show her their hairy legs at the follow-up clinics.

Thursday, 5th September 2013

What a difference a year makes. I am back to work today. This time last year I had returned to work after five years on and off. I had organised a child minder, bought new shoes and a notebook, had topped up my Oystercard and was ready for a new experience. Who knew, only four weeks later, we would receive the news that Andrew had cancer? Joseph told me it was leukaemia whilst I was on my own in one of our primary schools. In the last year I have been on the biggest rollercoaster life has thrown at me. I have seen, experienced and heard things I wouldn't wish on anyone. However, I have also met many truly inspiring people who are sharing the same cancer agonies. I have experienced untold kindness and reconnected with many more of you via Facebook. I have continued to work, with a lot of help and understanding from my boss, work-mates and family. I love my job; and the mental space it gives me away from the cancer world has been a huge factor in keeping me sane.

Monday, 9th September 2013
Andrew's reception teacher and teaching assistant have been for his home visit so I guess it must really be happening. I am ready, but I am not ready. I want him to go and have a happy time and make new friends, but I am anxious he will feel left behind, having missed almost a year of pre-school. I hope he doesn't have too much catching up to do.

Thursday, 12th September 2013
On Tuesday I visited a new nursery and, on seeing the busy children playing, nearly cried. I was thinking about the year Andrew has missed out on. The same happened today whilst I was visiting a new primary school. On their first day, the reception children looked so smart, little and happy. It is nearly Andrew's turn.

Sunday, 15th September 2013
My smiley boy is emerging from his steroid depression cocoon this morning. Hopefully he will be back to normal for school tomorrow. Five weeks until the next lot.

Monday, 16th September 2013
Exhale. Relax. Both children are at school. Andrew and all the children were whisked in quickly by his teacher. He had a huge smile on his face, so there was no time for either of us to feel sad. I am off to go shopping and have a coffee in Dulwich, to spend money and distract myself.

I picked Andrew up at midday, he was full of beans and talking ten to the dozen. He loved his morning at school. We had a lovely huge cuddle on pick up. I am so incredibly proud of him.

Tuesday, 17th September 2013

It was a great morning again at school for Andrew, despite a melt down over a book bag mix up at pick up. He had an afternoon nap and then the nurses came to access him for bloods. Dexamethasone week last week means his neutrophils are high at 1.6 - great. Clara however is struggling with the attention he is getting, probably more so now his information leaflet has gone out to everyone in the entire school.

Thursday, 26th September 2013

Today was the first full day of school for Andrew - followed by an hour of tennis after school. We didn't plan that well. Yesterday he wasn't keen on going; I think the permanency of it struck him (and me!). However once there, he was as happy as ever. He has been eating his packed lunches every day and playing with Clara at lunchtimes. They seem to be forming a new brother/sister bond born out of playing away from Mummy and Daddy for an hour a day. Lovely.

Monday, 23rd September 2013

The children are both at school. I have a day off, so I read with some children from Clara's class and now I am home for a coffee before lunch with a friend. I love it. I have increased my days at work to three this year. I am still working Thursday and Friday, but will now work on Tuesdays as well. We still aren't using a childminder, but we will make the childcare work between us, with some help from my parents who live nearby.

Friday, 27th September 2013

Macmillan coffee mornings have a whole new emotional meaning for me this year. This time last year I was a mum who liked a piece of cake with her coffee and any excuse would do. Who knew five days after last year's coffee morning I would become a mum to cancer? At our local hospital Andrew has the most wondrous paediatric Macmillan nurse called Cat, who has looked after all of us on our journey. To all of you who are hosting or going to a Macmillan coffee morning today - Enjoy your cake! http://coffee.macmillan.org.uk/

Sunday, 29th September 2013

I have been looking back through my photo uploads on Facebook as we need a few to print out for Andrew's 'All About Me' homework. I am totally amazed at how different Andrew looks with no hair. We were so used to it at the time I couldn't appreciate how ill and 'cancery' he must have looked to all of you.

Monday, 30th September 2013

A post to give clarity over the pre-school nasal flu vaccination:

It is correct the vaccine is live for twenty-one days. No one in Andrew's immediate family (i.e. people he would be living with or seeing for a prolonged time) should have it, but little people living near us, who he might see in the playground at school, are not a risk to him. Children being treated for cancer are still encouraged to attend nursery, for example. So Cath, Laila can have it, as we only see you for an hour or so a week, but we won't come and spend time with family at the weekend for twenty-one days afterwards.

Friday, 1st October 2013

We all have songs which define moments in our life. As we approach the 3rd October, when our lives changed forever, I remember how I listened to a song on a loop: Emile Sande's 'Read all about it'. It was made all the more emotional because a teenager from one of the Multi Academy Trust secondary academies sang it at a conference I attended at the end of October 2012.

We had this song and a few others on an album in the car and Clara and I would listen to the music a bit too loudly as we drove back and forth to the Queen Elizabeth or the Royal Marsden. Joseph would do exactly the same on the return journey. It kept Clara occupied; it gave us a release to rage and sing at the top of our voices.

Thursday, 3rd October 2013

I don't want the commission from this year's Usborne book order. I want to do something to keep myself busy and give you, my friends a way of helping. Please consider buying a book from www.usborne.com and take twenty-four percent off the price of any book.

Many people asked me a year ago "What can I do?" and told me to ask for help whenever I needed it. However, this needed a brainpower I didn't possess. I could organise myself back then. What I couldn't do was answer the question "what can I do?" I never knew how to answer in the moment. Which of the hundreds of jobs in my head could I delegate to someone else? I would smile and say thank you, say I would let them know if there was something they could do, but more often than not I did not.

We were lucky to have friends and family who 'just did it'. My next door neighbour cooked dinners, placed them in foil containers and stored them in our freezer. She had a key so let herself in. It was wonderful because, when we were at home we had a homemade meal to eat, including little portions for Clara. It meant we had a homemade meal to eat in the hospital too, when the tendency is to sit around and eat scraps of leftovers from Andrew's plate or fast food from the café. Other friends popped around with casseroles, bolognese, cake and wine.

One friend visited us one afternoon and arrived with a host of delicious foods from Marks and Spencer, some of which could be frozen. Another sent an Ocado order to our house, much to the confusion of the driver, who delivered two orders from the same van to the same house.

Keeping a routine for Clara was very important for Joseph and me. We would sacrifice our own sleep, and time with each other, to ensure Clara was content. We were grateful she was older than Andrew and at school already. My friends with daughters the same age would have Clara over at a moment's notice, any time of day, for a meal, fun and friendship. There were times when we overdid this. There were days when she screamed and shouted at us when we picked her up. She felt the abandonment, but we were doing the best we could and thought we were giving her the best opportunities we could in the circumstances. It was heartbreaking sometimes, as we couldn't get cross with her when she was getting mad with us. We waited for her to finish her rant and then cuddled her.

I remember once collecting her from a play date and wanting to drive home but she wanted to walk home. I got her in the car, but she wouldn't put her seat belt on. She was so cross and crying and shouting. I was exhausted and wanted to get home, but I couldn't drive without her having her seat belt done up. It was frustrating, but I had to climb into the back with her and calm her down.

Often when Andrew was in hospital with Joseph, Clara would sleep in bed with me at home. She needed and still needs the reassurance that we aren't going to disappear in the middle of the night and leave her. She sleeps with her foot touching me. Clara developed a love of French plaits a year ago. She would ask me to braid her hair in the morning. It made me stop multi-tasking and whizzing around. It made me stand still and dedicate time to her for ten minutes. I knew what she was doing, and even though, over time I got better and faster, I still took my time.

At diagnosis, Clara had moved into Year One. Andrew has the same teacher and teaching assistant in reception that Clara had. At parents' evening this teacher told us that, throughout Year One, Clara would walk up to her in the morning and tell her what she was having for lunch. The teacher would pretend to write it down on her register. It was a small gesture but one that moved us deeply. To know Clara had someone going over and above the pastoral care she needed in school to make her feel safe and secure brings tears to my eyes.

One December day in 2012, when Andrew was in hospital, I got home and found a Christmas wreath on our front door. A neighbour had made her own and decided to do one for us too. It was a show of Christmas that had not reached the inside of the house, as we had not yet had the chance to get a tree and decorate it, (I had however done most of my Christmas shopping online). Another friend knew an author so organised for him to send the children signed copies of his children's books. They arrived when Andrew was beginning to come out of his intense steroid fog. The children were thrilled to see their names hand written by a real author inside the books.

The joy of Facebook a year ago was the connection I made with friends when I was stuck in hospital. I debated whether to start a blog but decided against it because I craved the response and dialogue I received from people following a post. I loved and still love reading about what normal people are doing. Reading other people's posts keeps me distracted, and informed of events happening in the outside world. It is like having my own two-way news channel.

Friday, 4th October 2013
£317.70 of book orders in twenty-four hours - amazing! What a wonderful way to end Andrew's first full week of school.

Monday, 7th October 2013
£644. We have hit the magical £600, which means that for each donation, Usborne gives 60% of the money in free books to the Marsden. So £644 equals £386 worth of books WOW!

Wednesday, 9th October 2013

I am going to bed on £940.08 but will hopefully reach over £1000 in the next few days, which means I earn an extra 2% commission – or another £20 which I can spend on books for the hospital. Thanks everyone! You are incredible! And, of course, this means over £600 of free books!

Friday, 11th October 2013

It was Andrew's turn at school today to talk about the contents of his 'All About Me' box. He spoke proudly of his beads of courage and what each of the colours represents. He even showed his beads of courage to the head teacher and received a HUGE sticker from him. The teaching assistant had to leave the room because she was so overwhelmed hearing him talk. The beads are such a wonderful visual representation of the journey Andrew is on. Telling someone that Andrew has chemo every day is one thing, but seeing a string of beads with a hundred white chemo beads on it, somehow helps to put it into context.

Saturday, 12th October 2013

I am working out the numbers for Andrew's beads of courage so I can pick them up on Tuesday at the Royal Marsden. He has been on Maintenance for eighty-four days. He has had chemotherapy for sixty-one of those, has been neutropenic for twenty-three days, had twelve blood tests, fifteen days of steroids, and twenty-four days of an antibiotics, BUT he only visited a hospital three times AND he has started school.

Sunday, 13th October 2013

We are at the Queen Elizabeth Hospital because Andrew has a high temperature. His neutrophils have dropped to 0.3, so we have to stay for forty-eight hours to have IV antibiotics. My fault completely for counting up his beads yesterday!

Monday, 14th October 2013

Andrew was asleep at 9pm, up at 1:30am and wide awake until 4:30am when he had another temperature spike. He was given Calpol, but then he was sick so he was given paracetamol again. Finally, he slept. He is now awake and eating dry Frosties - excited to be able to go to the schoolroom later.

Clara is dressed up as a pirate for her literacy work today - exciting! She is so lucky to be having such a great Year Two at Balgowan Primary School. At times like these I am so grateful for the loving consistency of everyone around.

Andrew got hot again this afternoon so we won't be coming home until Wednesday afternoon at the earliest. He starts his steroids tomorrow. It will be hard to satisfy his cravings with hospital food. Joseph is at the hospital now so I can work tonight and tomorrow.

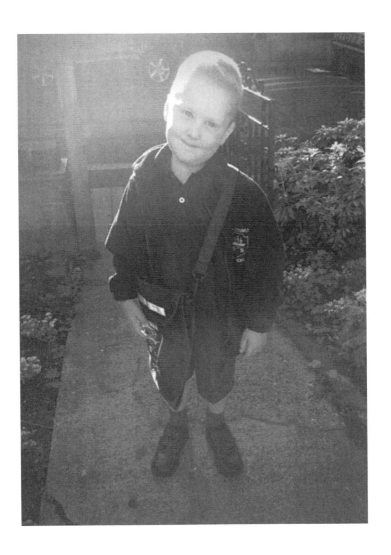

Chapter 9

Long Term Maintenance – Cycle 2

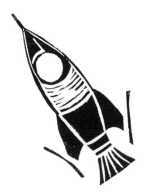

Four cancer winters

Full of colds, germs and worry

Hoping to stay well

Tuesday, 15th October 2013

Andrew's temperature was thirty-eight degrees at 2am so we will have to do another forty-eight hours from then. Annoying viral infections!

Wednesday, 16th October 2013

I am on the way back to the hospital to spend some time with my little boy. One more day and night and then maybe we can come home tomorrow.

There were lots of tears from Andrew when Clara and Daddy left the hospital to go home tonight; he wanted her to stay. It was heartbreaking to see them holding on to each other whilst he cried.

Thursday, 17th October 2013

Andrew is well enough to start Cycle Two of Maintenance and have his vincristine chemo and dex today. We are home now, though not yet through the front door due to the excitement of a frog on the front path. I love him. Despite everything that he is going through he is just a normal four year old boy.

£1398 equals £839 of free books for the hospitals – the order is going through tomorrow. Amazing!

Friday, 18th October 2013

I am blessed and so proud of Andrew who did his first day at school on steroids, and also of Clara who, in a week of turmoil at home, wrote a powerful pirate story and got a certificate in assembly from the head teacher.

Monday, 21ˢᵗ October 2013

Day 5 and the last day of steroids. Andrew is at school. Let's see how long he lasts!

Sunday, 27 October 2013

We have had a totally brilliant weekend at Legoland for Halloween horrors and fireworks fun. We treated ourselves to annual Merlin passes this year as we got a free adult carer pass. http://www.merlinmembership.co.uk/disabled. html. It might seem odd going to a theme park so much, but even if Andrew is neutropenic we can go and enjoy ourselves and seek out the thrills because we are outdoors and we fast track to the front of the queues.

Both children are now fast asleep in the car on the way home. It is half term and we have a week of general anaesthetics, with Clara's foot operation in the morning and Andrew's lumbar puncture on Thursday. Clara will be in bandages for a week, hence celebrating fireworks and Halloween this weekend. The middle toe on each of Clara's feet has always tucked under the adjacent toe. The doctors said they wouldn't do anything until she was five, so she is now having a small operation to cut the ligament at the base of each curled under toe. This will hopefully make the toe spring back into a straight position.

Wednesday, 30ᵗʰ October 2013

Thanks for all my birthday wishes. I have had a wonderful day, full of gorgeous presents and cards. Clara is up on her feet again. Her summer sandals fit over the bandages so she is enjoying herself walking around. She is certainly better, as she has returned to her usual, bossy self. An early night in order as all three of us are off to the Royal Marsden at 7:30am for Andrew's lumbar puncture, then home for pumpkin carving and Halloween fun. I am so looking forward to this week of hospital trips and operation recovery being over. I will be taking with me the three boxes of Usborne books which we are giving to the Royal Marsden children.

Thursday, 31st October 2013

Everything was easy and straight forward at the Royal Marsden, what a relief. We were home by midday - which is unheard of. Andrew is sleeping it off on the sofa whilst Clara and I make Hama bead Halloween shapes and catch up with Sophie Ellis Bextor on last weekend's 'Strictly Come Dancing.'

Tuesday, 5th November 2013

I have been to the dentist with the children and I have a dysfunctional jaw, e.g. clicking when I open it. It is caused by stress and the clenching and grinding of teeth. Go figure! It might explain my headaches too. I must find a way to relax.

Friday, 8th November 2013

There was a full scale meltdown on collecting the children after work today (them, not me), but boy was I grateful to be collecting them, (albeit screaming). We have now had one full week of not being stuck at home or in hospital. We are still taking each day as it comes and I'm grateful to come home at the end of the day together.

Sunday, 10th November 2013

The grotto at Intu Bromley are supporting Make a Wish Foundation this Christmas, so if you are passing, please pop a donation into their wishing well. Knowing we will be able to have a wish granted at the end of Andrew's cancer treatment by a wish-granting charity is keeping us going.

Wednesday, 13th November 2013

I am taking Andrew to the Queen Elizabeth Hospital for his monthly injected vincristine chemotherapy and to pick up dexamethasone. I am also dropping off the Usborne books. I am dreading the steroids again. To put it into context, the next five days following his vincristine chemo mean:

1. He gradually stops walking again due to leg pain and joint pain, and we have to carry him up and down the stairs and use the pushchair out and about
2. He needs codeine for his leg pain
3. He needs Movicol for constipation caused by chemotherapy and codeine
4. He gets thirsty so tends to drink a lot of water and also tends to have little 'accidents'
5. He has food cravings, like I had in the early stages of pregnancy, where he wants something but then doesn't want it and actually wants something else, which he then doesn't want… on repeat.
6. He gradually becomes lethargic and depressed so Clara loses her play partner
7. We have to sleep in with him as the depression makes him lonely in the middle of the night
8. He gets very tired and needs to sleep more, but the quality of sleep is less and he is wakeful in the night

Twenty-seven more months to go...

Thursday, 14th November 2013

We found out at Parents' Evening that Andrew is going to sing a duet in the nativity of 'Away in a Manger'. I am welling up already at the thought of it. Also his pen control is of concern, probably due to the vincristine chemo affecting the muscles in his hand and fingers. I had a guilty mummy moment when Clara told us her toe had been hurting all day and, upon taking her sock off, her left toe was swollen and infected. One swift trip to the emergency doctors later and we now have yucky antibiotics. Goodness me.

Friday, 15th November 2013

I have no interest in watching other 'Children in Need' tonight. I deal with enough sadness, day to day, without watching more on the TV - so I am planning a nice evening in front of 'Argo' with Joseph and a bottle of my favourite white wine.

Monday, 18th November 2013

And relax – Andrew's steroids are over for another month and they were extremely kind to us this time around - Andrew Bear is one super-duper amazing boy.

Wednesday, 20th November 2013

I am very touched as school asked me, this morning, which leukaemia charity they could support with a collection after the nativity. I thought it was our class but it applies for all three reception nativities. I chose the Royal Marsden Charity. That and Andrew's duet are going to make for an emotional morning! https://www.royalmarsden.org/

Friday, 22nd November 2013

Andrew asked me, at bedtime, after taking his daily chemotherapy, "Why do I still have to take medicine?"

I said, "So that you don't get poorly again," to which he replied, "There might be a war in my tummy."

It is the first time he has mentioned *still* having to take medicine.

Sunday, 24th November 2013

Wow, I have worked out, since Andrew was diagnosed with cancer, that I have raised £6710 for charities, through Usborne books, the Dryathlon, our Race for Life, the garden party, plus more from those who have raised money on our behalf, like a 19km run for CLIC Sargent and the Balgowan Primary School nativities to come. All of this money has gone, and will go, to the big charities like the Royal Marsden, Cancer Research and Macmillan. This is utterly unbelievable. Thank you.

I have decided that 2014 will be the year of fundraising for all the smaller charities who have supported us, like the Emily Ash Trust who gave us a week's respite holiday in August, Fatboys Charity who are sending us a very exciting present for Christmas, and Lucy's Days Out who arrange weekends away for families.

I am humbled by the people who set up charities to help others, day in day out. These charities offer big and small gestures, which mean such a lot to tired families like us on this long journey.

Monday, 25th November 2013

I am organising a short Santa Fun Run in the Recreational Ground in Beckenham, at 9:30am on Sunday 15th December - all money raised will be going towards local children's cancer charities. Santa hats a must. I was looking at the Santa Fun Run, which adults can take part in, in Bromley, but it is not for children, so I thought I would do my own! I have applied to the local council to see if I am allowed to have a group of children running around the paths.

Sunday, 8th December 2013

I have the official 'yes' from the local council - so long as we do not interfere with Sunday morning football, and stick to the paths near the café, we are allowed to do the Santa Fun Run - hooray! I have mapped out a route which is 1km long. Children can do one or two laps.

Wednesday, 11th December 2013

This month's vincristine chemo has wiped Andrew out. Today he slept for three hours in the afternoon - Day One of steroids done.

Thursday, 12th December 2013

This morning I had a flat tyre, a sick husband at home and a boy on steroids at Grandma's. How stressful. Andrew is not allowed to be anywhere near Daddy, for fear of catching his germs and ending up being admitted into hospital.

This afternoon the tyre is fixed; the husband is topped up with water, paracetamol/Ibuprofen and bread sticks at home; the Steroid Boy and Clara are asleep at Grandma's.

I am slightly less stressed, as I am in my pyjamas at Mum and Dad's, looking forward to a BIG glass of wine.

Friday, 13th December 2013

Wonder-Daddy is a lot better today and our Christmas tree is up. Steroid Boy is descending into a depressed fog and refusing to add any baubles to the Christmas tree, but still we soldier on. Confused Clara is not sure where her jolly playmate has gone. We made the mistake of mentioning to Andrew that Granny's dog, Kesia, might die soon as she is getting old. Now during steroid weeks Andrew lies awake at night worrying about her dying, "I don't want Kesia to die".

We are meeting up with family in the morning, then we are going to a pantomime in the afternoon. My Santa Fun Run is on Sunday morning and then we have an afternoon of loveliness with my new cancer family at the Emily Ash Trust's winter Wonderland. Can we do it? Yes, we can!

Sunday, 15th December 2013

The Santa Fun Run was a huge success and enjoyed by everyone involved, how thrilling! We had forty-two children come along, pay their £5 donation and run 1km or 2km around the park, wearing their Santa hats. Thanks to everyone who supported us by taking part. £340 raised so far. Fantastic!

Saturday, 21st December 2013

We received an iPad Mini today in the post, from the wonderful Fatboys Charity, and it has been hidden away. Many thanks. I have donated £250 from our children's Santa Fun Run towards their pot for next year's children.

I heard about this charity through the on line support groups. They fundraise all year long in order to buy children presents at Christmas. They have a network of people across the country who hand deliver the gifts to the child recipients. http://www.fatboyscharity.co.uk/

Monday, 23rd December 2013
Andrew's neutrophils have crashed; after five weeks of full dose mercaptopurine chemo, we are down to 0.4 and off all chemotherapy for a week. Never mind. Photos of Andrew this time last year remind us how poorly he was and how well he is now in comparison.

Wednesday, 25th December 2013
There was a moment about an hour ago when Andrew opened his iPad. He squealed like a little piggy! Thank you all so much, Fatboys. Merry Christmas to you all.

Tuesday, 31st December 2013
I have signed up for Cancer Research UK's Dryathlon again. I will be doing it in 2015 and 2016, before Andrew's chemotherapy ends on 20th February 2016. Joseph will be joining me too, so if you want to join the 4Andrew team let me know. I will be donating my wine money to my Dryathlon page especially as I already have three occasions booked in when I won't be able to drink. However, nothing will be as tough as January last year, when Andrew had his severe allergic reaction to platelets and was as swollen as a 'Spitting Image' character. There was a mini bottle of red in the food bag calling out to me then and I *really* needed to drink it but didn't.

Wednesday, 1st January 2014

We are in St. Osyth with Joseph's parents. We made it, despite Clara being sick in the car halfway up the A12. It was not remotely fun having to strip her off in the driving wind and rain on the side of the road. We also had to stop off at the Queen Elizabeth on the way because Andrew was complaining of an earache. I would quite like to go back to bed and start the day again!

Friday, 3rd January 2014

We are back home from the jaunt to Essex to see the Berthouds and Suffolk to see my parents. The last time we were at the latter it was the summer of 2012 and the London Olympics. Andrew was being a demanding three-year-old; he was six weeks off being diagnosed with cancer. It was great to go back and extend our comfort zone.

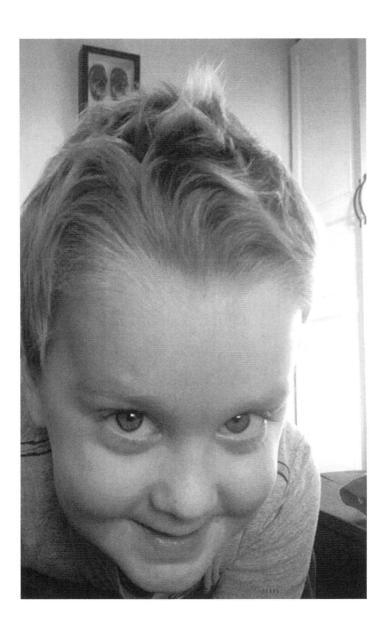

Chapter 10

Long Term Maintenance – Cycle 3

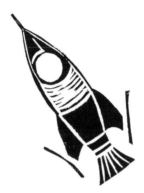

Good days help us get

Through the bad, sad and mad days

They go hand in hand

Tuesday, 7th January 2014

We are at the Royal Marsden Hospital this morning to start Cycle Three of Maintenance. It is very emotional coming back, and the visit brings memories of the early days. Even the smell of the soap in the toilets takes me back to the sluice room days. Andrew is content in the playroom, which makes up for missing the first day back to school. Observations have been done and he has no temperature, which is a relief.

We are at Queen Elizabeth Hospital now. Andrew had been back at school for fifty minutes when I got a phone call from the school office about a yellow discharge coming out of Andrew's ear. We are here now, getting it checked out. It is strange because he was checked over this morning by a doctor at the Royal Marsden and there was no mention of a sore ear.

Wednesday, 8th January 2014

Today my grumpy hungry caterpillar has emerged; he has eaten: one kiwi, one banana, one Pizza Express pizza (of course), one piece of toast with chocolate spread, one strawberry jam wrap, one bowl of cheerios, one Muller corner, one piece of chocolate cake, Weetabix, two cherry tomatoes, three strips of red pepper and nineteen different tablets for four different drugs. A fairly healthy day!

I collected Andrew's beads of courage this morning and have spent the evening threading them on. One thousand beads of courage in fourteen months of treatment. Twenty-five months left...

Saturday, 11th January 2014

Last steroid of the month done. Andrew has been pacing a lot today and has not been able to settle to anything; he is even dissatisfied with the TV or his iPad. He has eaten three tins of tuna just today. He is happiest bouncing outside in the fresh air on the trampoline.

Thursday, 16th January 2014

Yesterday I got a speeding fine through the door from 1st January, so I have the choice to do a speed awareness course. Today I have to abandon the car in Sydenham, as the gear box is making a funny noise in second and third gear. I am not a happy bunny!

Friday, 17th January 2014

The status report on the car is not great. We need a new gear box and clutch for about £3000. What an expensive start to 2014.

Saturday, 18th January 2014

Is it possible to feel even more fed up? I want to know who I have annoyed because karma is coming back to bite me. Today a parking fine plopped through the letter box! Bad news comes in threes for sure.

Monday, 20th January 2014

Great, bad news comes in fours... Now Andrew has a temperature of 39.3 so we have been admitted to Tiger Ward at the Queen Elizabeth.

Tuesday, 21st January 2014

Andrew's neutrophils are low at 0.2, so he has to stay in for forty-eight hours, having IV antibiotics. Joseph is with him and he feels ill now too. I am going home to pack a 'bag of fun' for my boys to keep them occupied. There have been no more temperatures since early this morning. Hopefully Andrew will be home on Thursday. We are due for a lumbar puncture at the Royal Marsden on Friday, but I am not sure if it will go ahead yet. During intense chemotherapy, we had a bag packed with some essentials – but we have got out of the habit now. Our essentials were:

- cheap batteries to replace the ones in the playroom toys, TV remote controls and Wii controllers
- McVities chocolate digestives
- Mini bottles of red wine - a bit naughty so a bit nice
- Chocolate Nesquik and cartons of Ribena – anything to help Andrew drink
- Mini boxes of cereal – the nurses often wake us up at 6am to do observations, but breakfast isn't until 8:30.
- iPad, charger and headphones – every Friday whilst at home I downloaded a set of programmes on BBC iPlayer, in case we were admitted into hospital and the TVs were not working
- Bedtime reading books – to try and keep routines as normal as possible
- A Tupperware pot of Lego bricks
- Toys which get Andrew out of bed – toy cars and a small ball
- Compact toys to pass the time – Snap, Top Trumps, Shut the Box or sticker books
- Playmobil characters – we have to wash our hands a lot in hospital and Andrew objects quite often, so instead, each time, we fill the basin with warm soapy water and give some of the people a bath

Wednesday, 22nd January 2014

Andrew's CRP infection marker has jumped to 160 overnight, 100 being normal for an ordinary infection, so we will be in for another night whilst we wait to see if something has been grown in the blood culture taken when Andrew first spiked a high temperature.

Suddenly my boys are in a cab, coming home. I wondered why until I saw Joseph who has a temperature of 39. I am not sure I can take any more of this! At least he is at home and not in the hospital so I can look after them.

Friday, 24th January 2014

Andrew is having a lumbar puncture at the Royal Marsden today. However, when the nurse did his observations on arrival they recorded his temperature as 38.9, so everything has been cancelled and we have to go back to the local hospital for the weekend. Give me strength. My resilience is being tested this week. Andrew has to be transferred to the Queen Elizabeth from the Royal Marsden by ambulance, with which means leaving my car in the car park and arriving with nothing at the Queen Elizabeth.

Saturday, 25th January 2014

Happy hospital Saturday! No high temperatures have been recorded since arriving at the Queen Elizabeth. The regular IV 'bleach' antibiotics seem to be helping. There are no remotes or batteries for our TV on the wall, but clever Daddy packed an aerial for the 'Starlight' TV shaped like a robot which can be wheeled between rooms. The journey to the Queen Elizabeth from the Royal Marsden almost directly passes our house. Last night the ambulance driver agreed, kindly, to make a stop so that Joseph could give us a bag of things we needed. It was very kind of the ambulance crew because it saved Joseph and Clara a return trip to see us.

Sunday, 26th January 2014

The rubbishness continues. We were all packed and ready to go home this morning, as the blood cultures had come back negative. Yet the Royal Marsden say we have to stay for another forty-eight hours, as Andrew had a temperature of 37.9 last night. No one told me. I spent ten minutes on the phone with a Doctor, arguing, but as his neutrophils have dropped from 0.4 to 0.2 overnight, stay we must. Another mum told the day nurse that her child had a temperature spike of 37.9 and it wasn't recorded on his chart; however, Andrew has a random 37.9 on his chart, so it appears there has been an error. I am waiting, with my still-packed bags, for the nurse from last night to get in touch to find out who spiked!

We are allowed home late this afternoon. Joseph and Andrew are both on antibiotics. Clara is running a temperature of 38.2 now, but we're home. Human error was identified and Andrew did not have a temperature of 37.9. Thank you to Dan for picking up the car from the Royal Marsden and driving it home, Mum and Dad for all sorts of taxi, food and Clara-related tasks, Cath for coming to see us today, Laila for the chocolate cake, and Lucas for the 'Star Wars' pictures.

Tuesday, 28th January 2014

And back we go to the local. Andrew has a temperature of 39.1. Silent scream.

Two and a half hours of sitting in traffic jams later, we have arrived. We missed dinner, but at least we have the same room and we have the Wii. Andrew's temperature was 38.2 on arrival. I am eating a microwaved Findus chicken curry for one bought from a local corner shop, whilst watching 'Power Rangers' and waiting for a portable X-ray of Andrew's chest.

Wednesday, 29th January 2014

I was up and out of hospital for an 8:30am meeting and left Andrew sleeping. Joseph taxied over to be with him. I am back now in hospital. Andrew's neutrophils today are 0.1. He has had no more temperatures, so we will be here until Friday morning if not longer. He is placated, painting for now. I am overwhelmed with tiredness.

Thursday, 30th January 2014

I have had a busy day at work but I am now back at the hospital with Andrew, who will hopefully be out in the morning. Enough now. Clara is sad and missing us. I have been busy telling her about all the nice treats we get because of Andrew's cancer. I told her to think about what the next nice treat might be. It is a hard concept for a six-year-old when all she wants is her mummy at home.

And tonight in my email inbox, the next nice thing...

Hi Andrew! My name is Camilla and I work for a charity called CFC – Cyclists Fighting Cancer – and the reason I'm writing to you is that, in November last year, I received an application, from your Mummy, for a bike award for you. I hope that the reason for my email might bring a smile to your face! Your bike application has been successful! We have decided that you should definitely have a brand new bike. We know that Clara already has a bike, but we are also going to give one to your Mummy and Daddy, so that you can all go cycling together! Your new bike will help you build up your strength and fitness and, of course, you can get out and about and have some fun! http://www.cyclistsfc.org.uk/

Friday, 31st January 2014
In, out. In, out. In, OUT! We are home.

Wednesday, 5th February 2014
We are at Queen Elizabeth Hospital, back for a spot of IV vincristine chemo. I exhaled when Andrew's temperature measured a normal 36.5. I wonder if I will ever stop holding my breath when his temperature is being measured.

We have also dropped off some brand new toys plus batteries. The beginning of some 'toy love' being passed their way, and hopefully the end of broken toys and hand-me-downs with missing pieces. This has all been paid for with the last of the Santa Fun Run money.

Saturday, 8th February 2014
Woohoo! Thanks to another generous donation, tonight, I have been able to buy *more* brand new toys for the oncology playroom at the Queen Elizabeth. I bought a big wooden dolls' house and dolls, a wipe-able car mat and cars, a toy microwave and Mega Bloks building bricks. They will be blown away.

Wednesday, 12th February 2014

We have had three weeks off all chemotherapy, but Andrew is starting again today, as his neutrophils have been boosted to 5.3 after steroids. I shall turn the alarm reminders on my phone back on.

Thursday, 13th February 2014

Andrew had a tantrum for twenty-five minutes because there were no courgettes in the lasagne I made for dinner. The last steroid was Monday morning!

Friday, 14th February 2014

I woke up at 2am, remembering I had given Andrew oral methotrexate chemo on Wednesday, meaning he couldn't have it again today in his lumbar puncture – so stupid! So the lumbar puncture was cancelled at 7am and postponed until Wednesday next week.

Wednesday, 19th February 2014

We are at the Royal Marsden Hospital for a half term lumbar puncture. Andrew's temperature is 36.5 - relax and exhale.

Thursday, 20th February 2014

Today in two years' time, it will be the end of our cancer journey – 20th February 2016. It started with lots of hard decisions. We decided some basics very early on, fuelled by being told "statistics show, if he was going to die, it would have been in the first ten days - they are vital." Staying together at home, as a family, is our priority and therefore we pass by on situations which put Andrew at risk of infection and will continue to do so. We won't travel too far from home, so that we don't end up in a strange hospital: so no far-flung holidays for another two years. We will enjoy each day as it comes and plan for the short-term future only. Not like the old me at all. We take advantage of all the 'nice' silver linings offered to us, where possible. Everything could change tomorrow; there is the chance Andrew could relapse and need a bone marrow transplant with months in hospital. Even at the end of our journey, the risk factors increase off-treatment. So we plod on, with the safety of our friends, family, routines, medicine and hospitals, to 20th February 2016.

Tuesday, 25th February 2014
There is suspected chickenpox in Andrew's class, so an extra blood test is needed today to see if he still has immunity after all the chemo. If it is chickenpox and he hasn't any immunity then he will be off school, waiting for a ZIG injection, which comes from King's College Hospital, London.

Thursday, 27th February 2014
There is another case of chickenpox in Year One at school, but the great news is Andrew's results show he still has immunity. If he touched a weeping pox spot he might get shingles, but I cannot imagine how that would happen. Woohoo! More good news!

Tuesday, 4th March 2014
One chirpy boy was taken to Tiger Ward this morning with some of the toys bought with the extra donation. Thank you. We are bracing ourselves to lose happy Andrew for a week. Steroids, be kind to us this month, please.

Wednesday, 5th March 2014

Evans Cycles asked me, a few weeks back, if I would be happy to be interviewed for an article about the bikes we received from them and Cyclists Fighting Cancer (CFC). Of course, I said yes! This is what they wrote:

We're proud to be working with Cyclists Fighting Cancer (CFC) to help children and their families battle cancer. The Berthouds received bikes in February and have been happily frolicking on two wheels ever since – the children enjoying the family activity, and parents being reminded of their first meeting, on a cycling holiday aged fifteen.

Andrew Berthoud, now four, was diagnosed with cancer in October 2012 – he takes daily oral chemo, and once a month has injections. The chemotherapy can make his legs achy and weak, and he sometimes finds walking tiring. Andrew's mum, Melody, explained the effect cycling had on her son, saying: "Children with cancer are often registered as disabled, and the treatment can result in flat feet and achy legs. I do have a special pushchair for him, but we try not to use it – Andrew has a scooter, so if we have to walk far, he often uses that."

Cycling, however, doesn't result in the same fatigue as walking, and she said: "He is absolutely fine cycling – the bike is the right size for him, and it is very light – he just whizzes along." The family of four, which includes Andrew, his six-year-old sister, Clara, mum, Melody and dad, Joseph, now all have bikes – three of which came through CFC – a Trek Jet, 16" with stabilizers, and two Trek hybrid's.

Melody said: "I found the charity though my community of cancer mummies on Facebook, I actually only applied for one bike, for Andrew – but they offered us four – one each. Clara already had a bike, so I asked for just three."

The family collected the bikes on the first day of the half-term break, and have been enjoying riding in their local park. Melody, who is a teacher trainer for a federation of schools, said: "In the past, we've walked over to the park for Clara to ride – now we all have bikes we can ride together. She has been so excited to have the whole family riding with her."

The family are planning future trips, and Joseph intends to ride to Greenwich with Clara in the summer – with Melody and Andrew joining them for sections along the way. On top of that, they are also planning an exciting weekend at Centre Parcs in May, where the bikes will feature heavily (don't anyone tell the children about that trip, as they still don't know!).

Melody hasn't ridden for a few years, but she and her husband met at a youth hostel when they were both on cycling holidays. She said: "It's been so nice to be back on a bike again, and the hybrid bike is so light. It's lovely to have something we can all enjoy as a family."

She added: "The application process with CFC was really simple, and everyone at Evans Cycles was so lovely. I'm really thankful."

Saturday, 8th March 2014

The last steroid of March has been taken. Twenty-three more months to go. For the majority of the day Andrew needed to be as close to me as possible and preferably cuddled tummy to tummy. I suppose it is a bit like when I used to carry him on my tummy in the sling, except he is considerably heavier.

Monday, 10th March 2014

I look at the three and four-year-old pre-schoolers running around the playground thinking about the year we missed, how I am not ever going to get back that time, and it makes me feel intensely sad. However, Andrew is every inch the normal nearly five-year-old in so many ways that it makes me grateful for what I have right now.

Thursday, 13th March 2014

I am so proud of my Andrew Bear who jumped into bed and read me a book this morning! Joseph and I are taking all the credit for Andrew learning his phonics and learning to read over the winter when we spent so much time in hospital.

Tuesday, 18th March 2014

Andrew is neutropenic - 0.4, so no chemotherapy for a week. It has been a while since we have had to be careful socialising. I am glad we found out after he and Joseph had been on public transport for a school trip to the London Transport Museum and not before.

Tuesday, 25th March 2014

Happy birthday to lovely Joseph. I was up early for a birthday breakfast so I could scoot off to Haringey to observe students and train newly-qualified teachers, then home again for mussels and chips for dinner (Clara too!) and a family game of Headbandz. The best present is probably that Andrew has some neutrophils, so is not immune-suppressed this week. It is two weeks until Clara is seven and five weeks until Andrew is five.

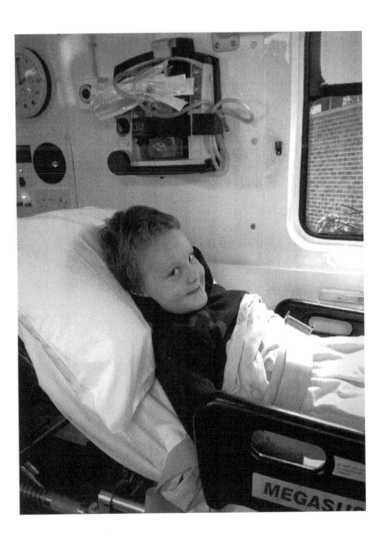

Chapter 11

Long Term Maintenance – Cycle 4

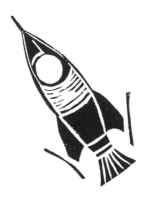

What if there were no

Cancer, where would we be now?

If the road forked right

Tuesday, 1ˢᵗ April 2014

What a quick three months! We are back at the Royal Marsden to start Cycle Four, with a consultant check-up, vincristine chemo and dexamethasone, steroids.

Cancer Mummies, Andrew has a school trip planned to a local farm. Should he go? Can he touch the animals? What would you do?

We regularly go to farms and pet the animals, as yet no bugs from animals!

No reason why not. Just make sure he is meticulous with hand-washing.

We went on a farm trip with school last year and it was fine. I gave my son a personal bottle of hand gel and his teacher made sure he washed his hands and used the gel at every opportunity.

Wednesday, 2ⁿᵈ April 2014

Walk away. Breathe. Count to ten. I HATE steroid week.

Thursday, 3ʳᵈ April 2014

Today I heard about a four-year-old who passed away because of cancer - I hate steroids, but I hate cancer more; at least I have my grumpy caterpillar at home with me.

Saturday, 5ᵗʰ April 2014

Andrew and I read Usborne's 'See Inside Your Body' book today. I used this book to explain leukaemia to Clara just after diagnosis. It was really fascinating and makes much more sense to me now.

Platelets clump around a cut. They trap red blood cells and form a scab. That is why a high number of platelets are needed for an invasive lumbar puncture and why Andrew's port continues to bleed if he has low platelets.

Red blood cells carry oxygen and take under a minute to travel around the body. Andrew was much more energetic and had colour in his cheeks after a blood transfusion because he was given more oxygen.

White blood cells hunt down germs that cause infections and gobble them up. Leukaemia derives from the Greek 'leukos' – 'white' and 'aima' – 'blood'. Leukaemia is all about the number or balance of white blood cells in blood. Children with Leukaemia have too many abnormal blast white cells being produced in the bone marrow, which then crowd out the generation of normal white cells

Neutrophils are a type of white blood cell and are the first cells on the scene when there is inflammation in the body. They don't last for long, which is why neutrophil levels can be deceivingly high just before Andrew gets ill. It explains why the blood count results phoned through each week are linked. The white blood count is normally slightly higher than the neutrophils. It also explains, when Andrew has low neutrophils, why he has nothing with which to fight the infection.

Wednesday, 16th April 2014

I am at the Royal Marsden Hospital with a hungry and thirsty four-year-old waiting for his lumbar puncture. I am glad Clara is here to distract us and he knows we will go to IKEA later for a post nil-by-mouth hunger pit stop - meatballs and chips.

Thursday, 17th April 2014
We had a great day with Cath and kids at Hever Castle. I got home and went straight to bed to sleep for an hour. I think my body knows that it is finally time for me to have a holiday; I have four days with Joseph and our families.

Friday, 18th April 2014
We are at the Round Table Easter egg hunt in the Recreation Ground. Another opportunity to say thanks to the Beckenham Round Table for buying Andrew's bed at the beginning of our cancer journey.

Thursday, 24th April 2014
I have had a fabulous day - I cannot believe my luck.

1. I have been asked to go on a work trip to Canada. I get to go on a plane!
2. I am in the process of trying to set up a Support Group and a local charity. The Chartwell Cancer Trust, who currently support adults in Bromley with cancer, want me to team up with them, their expertise and resources.

About four months into treatment, we were in the playroom at the Royal Marsden when I met another family. We got talking, and I discovered they lived in Farnborough, Kent. I was astounded, shocked and angry that there was another family, in Bromley, with a child undergoing cancer treatment, and that no one had told me within the four months since diagnosis. I thought we were the only family in Bromley with a child who had cancer and that realisation was isolating and frightening. I couldn't understand why the community nurses hadn't told me they treated other cancer patients in Bromley. I realise now they couldn't due to data protection, but at the time, I was bewildered. I also felt foolish because, of course, there must have been other families; we are not special.

Bromley families face a unique situation, as both hospitals we visit for treatment are outside the Bromley borough. If you are an adult, diagnosed with cancer in Bromley, you are treated at the Princess Royal University Hospital (PRUH) in Farnborough. However, all paediatric oncology, which used to be spread across two sites, was moved to the Queen Elizabeth in Woolwich at Easter, 2012. The Queen Elizabeth serves three London boroughs. Most of us also then go to the Royal Marsden Hospital in Sutton, which covers an even larger area.

I spent a long time being angry and cross, but then I felt sure there was something that could be done. I knew I must be able to set up some kind of support group for the families in Bromley; I didn't want anyone else to feel isolated and I want to reach out to people who live in Bromley. The Facebook ALL and Royal Marsden parent groups are very supportive, but it is not the same as talking face to face with people.

One evening last week I was driving to Biggin Hill to meet NCT friends for dinner and I passed by the airport. On the fence there was a poster for a fun walk, organised by a charity called the Chartwell Cancer Trust.

I have spent some time googling local leukaemia charities in the hope I could find financial support to establish a support group for Bromley families. Therefore, I was surprised there was a charity I had not heard of. When I got home I looked them up. It turned out the Chartwell Cancer Trust (CCT) - http://chartwellcancertrust.co.uk/ - are a registered charity, providing financial support for the Chartwell Cancer and Leukaemia Unit in the Princess Royal University Hospital (PRUH) for adults. Yet children are not treated at the PRUH so we cannot tap in to any of the support being offered to the adults.

I emailed the charity to explain about the children in Bromley and how I wanted to start a support group for these families. I wanted to know if they would be willing to contribute to the tea and coffee kitty and maybe the hall hire needed for the meet ups. My idea is to organise monthly meets in a neutropenia-friendly environment where families can talk, siblings can make friends and children with cancer can feel normal. When Michael phoned me today he said, "Yes!". What an amazing feeling!

Saturday, 26th April 2014
We had Andrew's birthday party today, a week early, as we are going to be at the Legoland Hotel next weekend - sssh, the children don't know - and Andrew had a special superhero fifth birthday party with the great Mr. Shillings. I put in a request for a cake with Baking a Smile - http://www.bakingasmile.org/ - and they found a local baker who was willing to meet my requirements and my party deadline for free. We had a beautiful hedgehog cake, covered in chocolate flake spines, from a baker called Becs.

Thursday, 1st May 2014

I was gazing, this morning, at gorgeous, snuggly Andrew who ended up in bed with me. I reached out to stroke him, woke him and then I realised he was a steroid monster: "Stop it, Mummy", "Go away". Half an hour later, he is painting farm animals in the kitchen.

Saturday, 3rd May 2014

Happy Fifth Birthday, Andrew. You've been through more life experiences than anyone should have at five years old. You are amazing, precious, awesome and an inspiration. We love you. Roll on, a well-deserved surprise 'Star Wars' weekend at Legoland with Cath, Dan, Lucas and Laila.

Saturday, 10th May 2014

For sale: one five-year-old who won't sleep past 6am.

Sunday, 11th May 2014

A massive thanks to Lucy's Days Out for our weekend in Centre Parcs. There was no signal, limited Wi-Fi, plenty of fresh air and an abundance of family time. The children have shimmied up a climbing wall, pony-trekked through the forest, thrashed us at ten pin bowling, thrown themselves down endless water slides, fired mini crossbows, zoomed on mini jet skis, played 10p slots to earn sweet money, cycled everywhere and shown no fear on an aerial adventure. I even managed to have a massage, sit down with a coffee to read a magazine and enjoy a beer with Joseph. We are thoroughly exhausted! http://www.lucysdaysout.org/

Saturday, 17th May 2014

We are at the Queen Elizabeth, getting Andrew's sore ear and conjunctivitis sorted out, after another night of practically no sleep. I should have brought toiletries for a shower, seeing as we have no hot water; instead we have water dripping through our bedroom ceiling.

Tuesday, 20th May 2014

I have been struggling with my own ear infections since Saturday, but I have just been given the all clear to fly to Toronto tomorrow. PHEW!

Sunday, 25th May 2014

All my interviews with Canadian teachers are completed. Yesterday we had a day off and drove to Niagara Falls, which was just incredible. On Friday night I drank cocktails on the fifty-first floor of a building at sunset. I have made thirteen offers in total to primary teachers wanting to come to London: fingers crossed some of them decide to relocate. I landed at 10.30am this morning after a night flight and was met at the airport by two squealing mini Berthouds. We are home now, enjoying a perfect rainy BBQ and Pimms. I get a week of half term fun with my two whilst fighting jet lag!

Wednesday, 28th May 2014

We are at the Queen Elizabeth for steroids. Whoop de doo.

Monday, 2nd June 2014

I have received a letter from Bromley telling me they are concerned about Andrew's weight; therefore, I need to get in touch with them as soon as possible - all because he was weighed at school on steroid week. I rang the nurse straight away and let her talk about her concerns of my son's obesity, then I said, "Are you aware my son has cancer?" It went very quiet at her end of the phone. Is it too much to ask for some linked up communication and thinking?

Saturday, 7th June 2014
We have received another letter about Andrew from our doctors' surgery; apparently he has not had his pre-school booster. Might it be because HE HAS CANCER? They diagnosed him. Surely THAT is on his records. I understand that the letters are randomly generated, but life with a child with cancer is stressful enough without having to spend time feeling upset and anxious about meaningless letters.

Sunday, 8th June 2014
Andrew is five centimetres taller than Clara was at the same age! Who says children on chemotherapy don't grow?!

Thursday, 12th June 2014
Today is exactly halfway through Andrew's treatment: twenty months done, twenty months to go. A great milestone to have reached. Every day now is closer to the end.

Sunday, 15th June 2014
I had a phone call from a doctor yesterday, which is unusual on a Saturday, asking to talk to me about Andrew's most recent blood work. Mind racing, heart in mouth, I listened, waiting to be told they had found blast (cancer) cells and Andrew was relapsing. Eventually she said nothing of the sort; rather she was ringing to talk about some mix

up over Andrew being very neutropenic, no one telling us the blood results for thirty-six hours, and thinking he was due IV vincristine chemo today. PHEW! Not a pleasant experience, despite the positive outcome.

Friday, 20th June 2014

In the 1960s, four percent of children with leukaemia survived. Now the survival figure is ninety-four percent - *that* is what research does; Clara has raised two hundred pounds for cancer research in anticipation of her Race for Life. Team Andrew is up to five hundred pounds!

Sunday, 22nd June 2014

I am bursting with pride as Clara AND Andrew completed the Race for Life at Crystal Palace today. Andrew walked 1km, then I pushed him the rest of the way in the McLaren pushchair, whilst Clara did the whole 5km, without moaning, in 55:20 minutes. A huge thanks and well done to Team Andrew! Six hundred and thirteen pounds raised.

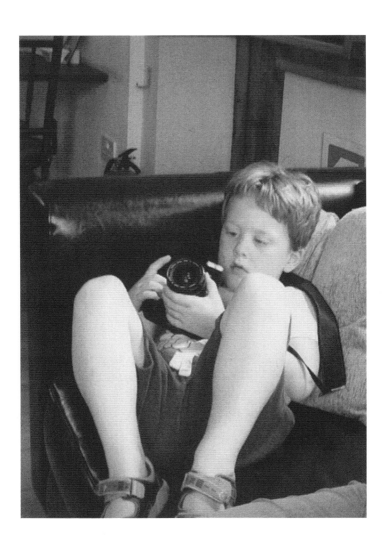

Chapter 12

Long Term Maintenance – Cycle 5

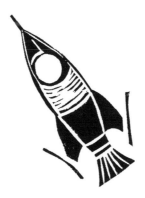

1 2 3 4 5

Dex monster is on the loose

6 7 8 9 10

Tuesday, 24th June 2014

Steroids and IV vincristine chemo always come around too fast. We are at the Royal Marsden, waiting to see our consultant for a three-monthly check up too. We are starting Cycle Five.

Friday, 27th June 2014

Today I went to the House of Commons to have lunch, courtesy of the Chartwell Cancer Trust. I was invited along to meet everyone and see the work that they do. I was very daunted, on my own, but it was amazing listening to the stories of fundraising that people have done for the charity.

Thursday, 3rd July 2014

I have all these photos on my phone of a bald kid who looks ill with cancer; I cannot believe it is Andrew. I didn't realise how the photos would look, for you out there, at the time it was happening. Stress protects and blinds us so we can carry on with our lives to ensure we don't crumple in a heap. I gain such comfort from seeing photos of those further ahead and hopefully there is some comfort brought for those at the beginning. Believe me, it passes soon enough, and one day you look back and think who is that?

Friday, 4th July 2014

Day One of 'Three Positives' Thanks for nominating me, Cath.

1.   Andrew's report was glowing: "A happy boy, full of fun, he has made good progress this year".

2. Clara's report was also full of praise: "She is a self-motivated learner and always tries her best," with great SATs results.
3. Andrew's attendance for the year is eighty-six percent, better than a lot of children not undergoing medical intervention.

Monday, 7th July 2014
Day Four of 'Three Positives'.

1. Andrew took part in his first sports day. He was too ill for the pre-school one last year.
2. Andrew came first in his obstacle race; he space-hopped over the finish line.
3. Clara got ten out of ten in her spelling test.

Tuesday, 8th July 2014 at 17:11
Day Five of 'Three Positives'.

1. Clara came second in the obstacle race and her house won the trophy.
2. We had a lovely classmate round for tea and a play-date with Andrew after school.
3. Andrew is first on the lumbar puncture list in the morning, so hopefully it will not be too long to wait with a nil-by-mouth child.

We seemed to have cracked Andrew waking up early only for it to be replaced by a Clara who cannot go to sleep and is often awake at nearly 9pm. I hope they don't join forces. It has been such a waste of an evening having to sit outside her door. Now Andrew is awake with a wavy feeling in his tummy - Lordy.

Wednesday, 9th July 2014

Some days there are storms; some days there are rainbows.

Today has been a stormy day. We were up at 5:45am for Andrew's twentieth general anaesthetic lumbar puncture at the Royal Marsden. We came home at midday and I was then at work until 11pm via Parents' Evening. As we were thinking about getting into bed, Andrew woke up and was sick everywhere.

Sunday, 13th July 2014

Rain. Lightning. Heavy rain. A river of water in the tent. Mud. Beer. Bacon. Sausages. Wet buns. Pastries. Coffee. Egg sarnies. Some sleep. Muddy children. Ambulance emergency (not an Andrew or a Berthoud). Forest fun. Football. Fox tail. Home. NAP! Lovely time at Epping Camp with the friends Joseph grew up with.

Monday, 14th July 2014

Today I decided Andrew had to write a sentence before he watched TV. He did this on his own and totally shocked me: "When we got to where our dad was, we went camping. I loved the marshmallows." Pretty amazing for a reluctant writer. I am very proud of him.

Tuesday, 22nd July 2014

We had a blast from the past today, at an appointment after school at the Queen Elizabeth for vincristine and dexamethasone. The nurse checking chemotherapy was the same as on that first day, when I had to restrain Andrew whilst the nurses tried to get a cannula into his little veins; up popped Mick with a glove balloon face. In the twenty-one months since we have talked about the balloon often and I've never managed to make one. Now we have two! Small things.

Wednesday, 23rd July 2014

One. Two. Three. Four. Five. Six. Seven. Eight. Nine. Ten. The dex monster on the loose. Mummy is hiding and counting to ten.

Knowing what food to give Andrew during steroid week is often a struggle. It is never the same. During the initial steroid block, he craved cheese and bread, and would devour cheese baguettes, cheesy Doritos, Quavers, pizzas and lasagne. The combination of vincristine and dexamethasone makes Andrew constipated, so making sure he eats healthily is a driving factor for his intake. It only took one month of letting Andrew eat what he wanted, when he wanted, and the excruciating constipation which followed to know we couldn't do it again.

Steroid week lasts for five days and, as the days go on, Andrew's desire to eat salad, vegetables or savoury food lessens, in favour of sweeter fruit or chocolate cake, chocolate in a wrap, or chocolate milk.

His taste buds change from month to month and week to week. He would eat curry in Early Maintenance but not now. He also has an acute sense of smell, so even the smell of pasta with butter makes him run out of the kitchen gagging. He liked my fish pie for a few months and then hated it; same with spaghetti bolognese too. It is so frustrating, but we do not cook him separate dinners. He has to try some of the food I prepare in order to earn something else. The 'something else' is an easy option e.g.

a bowl of cereal or a sandwich, and he has to have his five fresh fruit or vegetables a day.

There are some constants. He loves cereal (the sweeter the better), baked beans (they contain sugar of course), scrambled eggs (with ketchup, which is again sugary), French bread or Pizza Express Margherita, (but not the shop-bought ones which have herbs and pepper on them).

We stock up on the following foods:
> Sweeter vegetables and fruit:
> Red and yellow pepper (dipped in hummus or salad cream)
> Bananas
> Kiwis
> Grapes
> Pineapple
> Pears (dipped in melted chocolate)

We have scotch pancakes for breakfast at the weekend, so he eats lots of fruit AND the chocolate he craves, or we have fruit kebabs and he chooses the pattern of fruit.
Snacks with fibre:
> Go Ahead apple biscuits
> Malt loaf bars
> Weetabix – with a banana
> Shreddies – with a banana

By Day Five we are thrilled if he eats dried fruits such as:
> Raisins
> Dried apricots
> Yo Yos

Clara hates steroid week. Each month we tell her it is coming and warn her this is Andrew's grumpy week, but there is always a point where we have to remind her to ignore Andrew's mood and not react to it. She gets sulky and strops about saying "you didn't tell me" or "I forgot". She finds the injustice hard. Andrew is allowed to watch more TV so I can spend quality time with her; he is allowed to eat different dinners to us but when she tries to refuse food, she isn't allowed to. He is excused rudeness or moodiness, unlike her, because 'it isn't Andrew, it is the medicine; he cannot help it.'

We tell her off for provoking Andrew, or reacting to make him cross, but she doesn't understand. She loses her playmate for a week a month, and it always takes a few more days for her to get over the hurt and trust him enough to play with him again. By the end of the five days, the clingier Andrew gets and the more demanding Clara becomes. I have occasions where they are both fighting to sit next to me at dinner, or on the sofa, or to hold my hand. I arrange play-dates for her after school in steroid week, which she enjoys, but they probably perpetuate the abandonment she feels.

Joseph is mentally stronger during steroid week; he is so good at distracting Andrew and playing games with him. I retreat mentally, as I find it harder to deal with Andrew's moods. He is very Mummy-obsessed: he wants to cuddle me, sleep in bed with me, sit with me, hold my hand, stroke me or be stroked by me. The more he demands me and the more Clara needs me, the more I want to escape, as I feel so claustrophobic. I spend a lot of the week feeling guilty.

Friday, 25th July 2014

I am keeping it together by feeding the dex monster and Clara an early lunch at Pret a Manger.

Sunday, 27th July 2014

Happy Twelfth Anniversary, Mr Berthoud. Getting stronger every year, despite what life throws at us.

Monday, 4th August 2014

The Berthouds are on holiday enjoying sandcastles, sea, sand, Punch and Judy, ice creams and a bit of sun at Swanage beach.

Tuesday, August 5th 2014

Even though we are on holiday in Swanage, Andrew still needs a weekly blood test. We caught a little ferry across the water to Poole Hospital. There are lots of friendly nurses here. They have a parents' kitchen, so I am drinking coffee whilst the children play. It is interesting to see the provision in other hospitals, but I am glad this is only a quick visit.

Wednesday, August 6th 2014

We spent the day at Corfe Castle today. Andrew and I got the steam train past fields of campers and cows. Joseph and Clara walked the four miles from Swanage to meet us for a picnic lunch.

Friday, August 8th 2014

We have stopped for a quick cup of tea in Southampton with the children's godparents, to break up the journey home from Camp Bestival in Lulworth Cove and Swanage, then we are going on to spend a few days in Suffolk.

Yet more fun days to be had at Southwold beach and Bewilderwood.

Wednesday, August 13th 2014

I have already had a delicious crab lunch in Walberswick, Suffolk, and now I am trying to catch crabs with Andrew and Mum, whilst the rest of the family do a three mile walk.

Thursday, August 14th 2014

It is our last day in Suffolk. Now we are going on to Telford Fest, which Andrew and I missed last year, whilst he was on intensive chemotherapy. We are camping with Joseph's side of the family, all the aunts, uncles, cousins and second cousins. I can't wait!

Monday, August 18th 2014

Joseph and Andrew are at the Queen Elizabeth in Woolwich, as it is vincristine and steroid time again. Clara and I are eating cake with a hot chocolate at Buckingham Palace, having completed a tour of the state rooms, thanks to a birthday present from Grandma. Clara's hot chocolate has a chocolate crown dusted on the top. I think she was disappointed not to be able to go into the Queen's bedroom; I think she was hoping to be able to see her bed!

Wednesday, 20th August 2014

Eighteen months of chemo left today. 20th February 2016 – there is a small light at the end of the tunnel.

We have come to Gambados soft play in Beckenham. We are here early to beat the rush.

Steroid Andrew:	"Is it lunch time?"
	"No."
Andrew:	"Is it elevenses?"
	"No."
Andrew:	"What's the time?"
	"9.57am."
Andrew:	"Can I have tenses?"
	"No!"

Friday, 22nd August 2014

If I achieve nothing else all day on day Four of steroids, I have bought the kids' school shoes.

Sunday, 24th August 2014

Andrew is gradually returning to us today, now that the steroids are leaving his system.

Monday, 1st September 2014

Today is the beginning of Childhood Cancer Awareness month. In the UK, 2.5 million people are living with cancer. 1000 new people join every day. Around three thousand six hundred children and young people under twenty-five are diagnosed with cancer every year. In children under fifteen the most common type of cancer is leukaemia.

Tuesday, 2nd September 2014

There are some days where I can almost forget Andrew is being treated for cancer; he is so incredible in so many ways and so 'normal' too. My Facebook feed is filled with reminders, at the moment, of how wonderfully brave he is, how brave Clara is, we are, all the children, parents and siblings are, and more reminders of how utterly frightening, overwhelming and depressing it all is. Did I really go through that?

I am constantly grateful for another great day with my children and family, another day at work, another night where we are all together. Then a mum I know from back in those dark, dark early days, who gave us support, kindness and advice, found out that her daughter, a year off treatment, has relapsed. The threat is always there; it never leaves me. It will never leave me. We'll get to the end of Andrew's treatment - seventeen months' tomorrow – and I will still worry. He won't get the all clear for another five years after treatment finishes, which will be February 2021. We shed a tear for the family last night, but know somehow they will find the strength to be brave and strong all over again.

"If you ever see a child face cancer, it will change your life forever."

Wednesday, 3rd September 2014
Clara and Andrew are all set to go back to school and begin Year One and Year Three. How time flies!

We juggle our need to work with our desire to keep Andrew at home. Both our jobs can be computer-based, meaning we can more or less work anywhere, anytime. I have work emails on my home phone: a trade-off for the flexibility work gives me because we cannot send Andrew to fulltime childcare.

In January 2014 I was asked to take over the running of the Initial Teacher Training Programme for an extra fourth day a week. To help juggle the childcare, Joseph decreased his time to four days too. We share the school runs and, one day a week, we have help from my parents and a neighbour who is a childminder.

Monday, 8th September 2014

Four sleepy Berthouds are back together under one roof. Joseph and I have had a lovely, and much-needed, child-free weekend away in Malta. We woke up when we wanted, sat in the sun, read books, had siestas, ate dinner late at night and didn't worry about cancer or the children once. It was marvellous.

Friday, 12th September 2014

I am a proud Mummy, as Clara got a certificate in assembly and Andrew was chosen to have the class bear for the weekend. That, and a payrise, means, all in all, it has been a great day!

Saturday, 13th September 2014

A huge thanks to Children with Cancer UK and Zippo's Circus for a terrific time today in Peckham. The Horses, Hercules, Norman Barrett with his Budgies and the Tropicana Troupe were our highlights! Thanks also for the constant supply of food and drinks and a gift from the Entertainer at the end. It was an honour to be able to thank Mr Zippo himself. http://www.childrenwithcancer.org.uk/

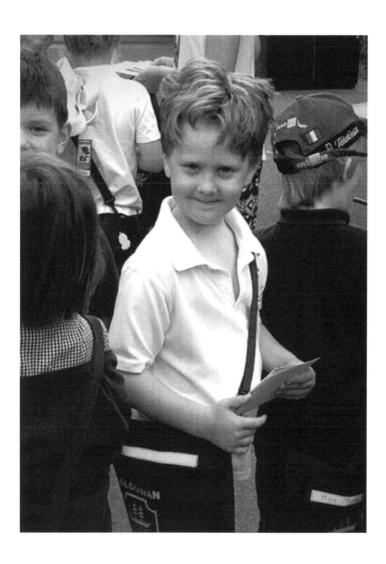

Chapter 13

Long Term Maintenance – Cycle 6

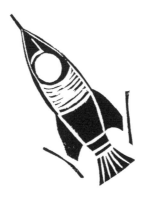

Diagnosis day

Is etched in my memories

Forever, always

Tuesday, 16th September 2014

Andrew is still in remission. What a wonderful sentence to hear. Another twelve weeks done; another course of steroids started. We are now on Cycle Six of twelve. It was wonderful to see friendly faces. Keep going. Keep strong.

Friday, 19th September 2014

I had a great day delivering the National College's Senior Leader training to senior staff in secondary and primary schools. I was very nervous at first but loved it. It is hard to remember sometimes that I am not just a mummy, and a cancer mummy, but I was a deputy head and an acting head in a past life.

Tuesday, 23rd September 2014

Andrew's neutrophils are high after a week of steroids (3.5), which is great because he has a cold, with a cough and runny nose. All perfectly normal for any five-year-old but stressful in a child being treated for cancer.

Thursday, 2nd October 2014

On this day two years ago, I noticed that Andrew had a fluid-filled spot on his tummy and thought that he had picked up chickenpox from pre-school, which would explain why he had been feeling so poorly. I dropped Clara off at school and drove around to Mum and Dad's house to seek their advice. Mum agreed it looked like the queen spot, so I rang the GP and asked for an appointment. It would have been the second time he had contracted chickenpox, which wasn't unheard of - I had chickenpox twice, and shingles, before I was eleven - but it was unusual.

As soon as we walked into the room, the GP, Dr. Navarro, asked me how long he had been pale for. "A while," I replied and told her that my friends had commented on it recently. She asked me if there was anything else wrong and I explained Andrew had been sick on Saturday night, had had nosebleeds, achy legs and lethargy. She wanted to give me some topical cream for the spot, which she decided wasn't chickenpox. She suggested I also take Andrew for a blood test to see why he was so pale. As soon as she said that, and after reeling off all the symptoms, I knew it could mean leukaemia.

So Mum came with us to Queen Mary's Hospital in Sidcup, where Andrew was given four patches of magic cream, one on each hand and foot. The doctors were obsessing over two bruises on his shins. Trying to get a cannula in to take blood out was utterly horrific. I pinned him against me whilst he screamed. I cried and Mum stroked me and they tried and failed repeatedly.

Then they succeeded and we waited. I had googled the symptoms of leukaemia before picking Mum up, so tentatively said I was worried it might be that. They wouldn't let us go until the results came back, but by 6pm when the clinic closed, there were still no results and we left and came home.

I voiced my fears to Joseph that night and, even though some Leukaemia symptoms fitted, others, such as 'excessive weight loss' and 'excessive bruising,' did not; so we talked ourselves out of it and went to sleep.

Friday, 3rd October 2014

On this day two years ago the spot on Andrew's tummy had ballooned overnight and the skin around it was inflamed. Joseph stayed at home with Andrew. Mid-morning, he was rung, told to pack an overnight bag and go to Hippo Ward at the Queen Elizabeth in Woolwich. The reason given was something to do with a high number of white blood cells. The bloods had only just been processed that morning despite being marked urgent yesterday.

Mum drove them in, as I had the car at work. The next thing I knew, Joseph phoned me to say I needed to come to the hospital. I asked why, and put Joseph in the difficult position of having to tell me what he had been told, knowing I was on my own and had to drive the twenty miles to the hospital. He didn't respond, so I asked, "Is it leukaemia?" His pause was enough.

The oncology consultant knelt down behind the bed, where Andrew was beginning his love affair with Apple products, and said, "We have found blast cells in Andrew's blood; we think it's leukaemia, which is eminently curable."

I left straight away, mind reeling. I remember phoning my boss and leaving a message. I was only four weeks into a new job. I don't remember much about the drive over the Dartford Bridge. I know I was shaking when I stopped at McDonalds for a break. When I arrived on the oncology ward, I had to face the reality: "The treatment will take three years; don't spoil him." No one had mentioned the C word yet. It was only when talk turned to finding us a bed at the Royal Marsden, which I knew was a cancer hospital, that I realised what that meant.

Andrew had to go through the horror of cannulas again, in order to be on fluids and blood immediately. Joseph held him tightly whilst the play specialists tried to distract him by blowing bubbles whilst we sang songs. Joseph worked through his repertoire of nursery rhymes but we both stopped mid-sentence when singing 'You are my Sunshine'. Suddenly we didn't want to face the reality of a world with our sunshine being taken away.

I then had to leave the boys to get five-year-old, Clara from school and try to explain where Andrew and Daddy had gone.

Saturday, 4th October 2014

Now that the deeply held memories of 3rd October 2012 have passed, I feel I can look forward to our third anniversary, when we will have only four months of treatment left - woohoo! Yesterday the founder of the Chartwell Cancer Trust rang me to say that they will continue to pay for all the costs of my monthly Bromley Childhood Cancer Support Group (BCCSG) meet ups. Moving forward, when the Berthouds are ready to leave cancer behind us and 'get on with our lives,' they will take over the running and organisation of BCCSG and it can be my legacy.

Two weeks after diagnosis I decided to do my annual Usborne Books at Home and School order, where all the books customers bought were reduced by twenty-four percent (my commission discount) and the collective total equated to free books. In the first year, the Royal Marsden received five hundred and fifty pounds' worth of free books; last year, when we did it, they received eight hundred pounds in free books. I would like to do it again this year; I will give the free books to The Royal Marsden, for the play team to use as Christmas presents, birthday presents and distraction presents, which they find invaluable. However, I am also going to use the free books to give each child going through cancer in Bromley, and their siblings, a present at Christmas time.

Wednesday, 8th October 2014

Home sweet home, after three nights and three days in Sheffield to learn how to deliver the Outstanding Teacher Programme. I came home to Andrew, who is fast asleep wearing a penguin hat, pyjamas and one sock, and a beautiful snoring Clara. I missed Mr. B and the mini Berthouds.

Friday, 10th October 2014

Two happy five-year-old superheroes are on the trampoline and two happy, bossy seven-year-olds are playing teachers upstairs. One mummy is getting lots of work done; I love play-dates. Our childcare arrangement means the children can go to after-school clubs and have play-dates. We can also have friends over to us for tea. Working four days a week means Joseph and I both have one day a week flexibility, for hospital appointments, without having to ask for time off. Every week is different. Joseph works either at the office or at home, but I have multiple places I have to be. We have a shared Google calendar, so we start the week by deciding who will pick up and drop off each day, but invariably it changes depending on meetings which crop up along the way.

Tuesday, 14th October 2014

Andrew's neutrophils are 0.2; they've not been low for ages and ages. This means a week off all chemotherapy and extra precautions so he does not catch an infection, which will land us in hospital. At least we have boosting steroids this week!

Thursday, 16th October 2014

Today is Andrew's first time off school due to steroids. He came home at lunch needing to sleep.

Monday, 20th October 2014

We are at the Queen Elizabeth getting Andrew checked out due to the croupy cough and a sore ear. He seems to end up with a viral croupy cough often and the cough signifies he is neutropenic. He has antibiotics for an ear infection and 0.0 neutrophils.

Thursday, 23rd October 2014

A high temperature at 4am means that Andrew is now lying in bed at the Queen Elizabeth at 6am, waiting to see a doctor. Boo. Neutrophils 0.1, CRP 43, so we need to wait forty-eight hours for blood cultures. It has been nine months since our last stay here!

We send Andrew in to school even with low neutrophils of 0.1 or 0.2. The school ring us regularly about chickenpox and other viruses that are going around. The leaflets, which were sent home to all new-starters, mean families are informed about phoning in illnesses. It is only when the illness concerns a friend Andrew plays with or sits next to that we worry and ask for the immunity check. We are lucky, as each time he has been tested, the results have come back showing he still has immunity. If his neutrophils are 0.0 however, like recently, then we don't send him in to school for fear of ending up in the Queen Elizabeth again and splitting up the family.

Andrew is so frequently sick in the night that, if we are sure it is chemotherapy-related sickness, we still send him to school. He is missing so much school anyway, for appointments or inpatient stays, so we want him to go as often as possible. If there is a school trip being planned, we ask the teachers, to avoid steroid weeks if possible. One or other of us will ensure we are free on the day, to accompany Andrew.

Friday, 24th October 2014
Many weeks of work and organisation have gone into today's three conferences, for over six hundred staff on three different sites. It has been made even harder because Andrew has been poorly this week. He's still coughing but has no temperature, so we are on course for coming home in the morning.

Saturday, 25th October 2014
Thank you, sunshine. My neutropenic boy is home and happy at the park, playing in the fresh air.

Thursday, 30th October 2014
Thanks for all the birthday wishes. I am having a lovely day. We got the piano tuned and Clara's flu jab done. We had a yummy lunch with mojitos at Jamie's Italian in Greenwich and now we're having a wander around the market.

Friday 31st October 2014

The Usborne book order has been placed! Many thanks to everyone who ordered books. The combined total of orders meant I was able to select four hundred and fifty pounds' worth of books for children with cancer.

Friday, 7th November 2014

Today is the first week in ages where I get to have my day off. Birthday vouchers = massage + haircut. Heaven.

Sunday 9th November 2014

I am organising another Santa Fun Run for children. Five pounds per child, with proceeds going to Bromley's Chartwell Cancer Trust who are helping me establish a Bromley Support Group: http://chartwellcancertrust. co.uk/

Children can complete 1km (one lap) or 2km (two laps) around the park. Bring your own Santa hat! There will be a certificate and prize for all who take part.

Monday, 10th November 2014

Poorly Clara is asleep on the sofa. It is stressful when the non-cancer child is sick. It frightens me. I didn't know Andrew's illnesses meant he had cancer, so would I know if it happened to Clara too? Would we be that unfortunate?

Tuesday, 11th November 2014

What would make a busy working week and a poorly Clara more fun? Steroids of course! Fifteen more to go...

Friday, 14ᵗʰ November 2014

Cancer Mummies: Andrew's fine motor control is a slight cause for concern e.g. pencil grip, control. His school are not sure if he can't do it due to the chemotherapy or isn't very good at writing! He did miss a whole year of pre-school, and isn't one for colouring. Has anyone else had similar problems with four-year-olds and writing?

Funny you should post this, as my son's teacher mentioned his weak grip at Parents' Evening. He's in Year One now and it wasn't a problem in reception, so I think it is the drugs. His writing was always quite good. He hasn't been affected in any other way by vincristine, so I think it's weak muscle from the steroids, as he had severe muscle wastage during induction. She recommended dot-to-dots and maze puzzles to improve his control.

My son couldn't do up buttons, use scissors or write. This was when he was four. Now at eight, he finally does it all beautifully. Wait till vincristine is over and you are off treatment, then work on it.

Sunday, 23ʳᵈ November 2014

It was lovely to see all the local cancer families this morning at Cafe Dolce Vita – in Petts Wood. It is a great venue, with delicious food and fantastic company. Thanks too to the Chartwell Cancer Trust for enabling it to happen.

When Michael Douglas, the founder and trustee of CCT rang me and said those magical words, "I want to help," I set about googling venues in the centre of Bromley which were available on Sunday mornings. Most churches had halls, but none were free on a Sunday morning.

I arranged the first meet up during August 2014, to be held in Kelsey Park, Beckenham, as it was the summer and even neutropenic children can be out in the fresh air. Three families came along. The next few meet ups were nonstarters, for various reasons. Probably because it was autumn and there were a lot of germs about. It was still difficult to get a regular venue and to think of an idea, which would suit children on treatment and their siblings, whilst also enabling parents to talk. A mum from the group told me about a café in Petts Wood which offered a private hire for us on a Sunday morning and it had a children's play corner. It sounded perfect.

I rang Café Dolce Vita and booked a Sunday morning. We had six families come along today and we all hit it off straight away. I brought along an assortment of arts and crafts activities for the children and they spent most of the time playing nicely whilst the parents chatted. The children were given sandwich boxes for lunch and we ate cake. It feels like the BCCSG has been properly formed.

Monday, 24th November 2014
We had a phone call about chickenpox in Andrew's class, but luckily after being tested again Andrew still has immunity - yippee!

Saturday, 6th December 2014
We were treated this afternoon, by the Chartwell Cancer Trust, to a pantomime at the Churchill Theatre, with a meet and greet from the main characters who gave the children presents afterwards. I was particularly pleased with a hug from 1980s pop star, Sonia!

However, we are now at the Queen Elizabeth with Andrew who coughed throughout. Andrew's temperature is 39.5. Neutrophils 1.8, CRP 20. He has had a throat swab and a chest X-ray. The Royal Marsden have been informed and we wait for protocol.

Sunday, 7th December 2014

Andrew's temperature is 37.8 this morning; no fluids needed as his temperature responded to Calpol. He slept well too. I had a lovely chat this morning with him on the phone and he only coughed once in ten minutes. He was disappointed to be missing the Santa Fun Run AND the Emily Ash Trust Winter Wonderland today. I am constantly amazed at the resilience of my children. I couldn't ask for anything more.

Thank you to everyone who came to the Santa Fun Run in the park this morning to run. We raised two hundred and thirty-five for The Chartwell Cancer Trust.

Andrew had another spike of 39 degrees this afternoon and a drop of neutrophils to 0.4. Boo. He didn't even want to eat his advent calendar chocolate; he MUST be ill!

We had another fabulous afternoon with so many of my favourite people and their children looking so well, thanks to the Emily Ash Trust. Clara had a wonderful afternoon, meeting Father Christmas and cuddling all the animals. She has fallen in love with a bunny rabbit called Harvey. Thank you for our vouchers and the goody bag of arts and crafts for Andrew; it is such a shame he missed out.

Monday, 8th December 2014

I am so relieved as Andrew is coming home with a big bag of drugs! His neutrophils are 1.3 and there have been no temperatures for twenty-four hours. He has been given oral antibiotics for the cough and antibiotic drops for an ear infection.

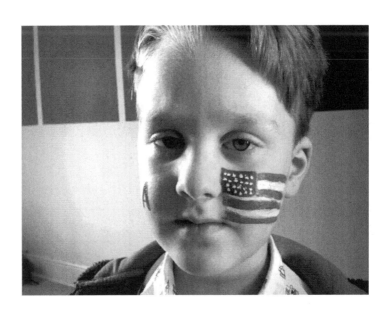

Chapter 14

Long Term Maintenance – Cycle 7

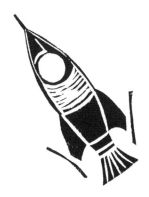

It's like being on

A rocket to the moon

You cannot get off

Tuesday, 9th December 2014

It is the vincristine and dexamethasone time of the month at the Royal Marsden for the start of Cycle Seven. I picked up six months' worth of beads of courage and dropped off this year's Usborne books to the play team too. Another three months done: another three months in remission and cancer free. Steroids of course meant Pizza Express for lunch. At 5pm Clara was brought back from a play date and screamed for thirty minutes, "My ear, my ear!" One emergency doctor appointment later, she also has antibiotics for an ear infection. I am surprised the GP didn't prescribe me a course of red wine.

Thursday, 11th December 2014

Day Seven Hundred and Ninety-Nine of treatment. Bead update: Andrew has approximately one thousand seven hundred and fifty beads of courage. Cancer, we're winning and there's proof!

The beads are issued by Be Child Cancer Aware. They train hospitals in the Beads of Courage programme and issue the beads of courage in the UK. They run competitions through their Facebook group for additional special beads. We have made Andrew's beads into the shape of a spider, teddy bear, a letter A, a heart and a sunshine to win beads. They ran another competition where we had to make our beads into the shape of a building, which could be lit up in September for 'Go Gold for Childhood Cancer'. We recreated the London eye. I also bought a sibling pack of beads from them to give to Clara in the early days. It meant she could collect beads for special events, such as being moved from pillar to post or sometimes going to school not knowing who would pick her up: http://www. bechildcanceraware.org/

Friday, 12th December 2014
Today is the last dexamethasone of 2014... Woohoo! Merry Christmas! Fourteen more months to go.

Saturday, 13th December 2014
We are all at the Royal Albert Hall, feeling very proud whilst watching Joseph sing his heart out up on stage. I had to apologise to everyone sat around us as Andrew coughed most of the way through the concert, before falling asleep on me. Clara stood up and sang 'Away in a Manger' with all the other children in the hall – she is marvellous!

Sunday, 14th December 2014
Andrew and Clara are playing...together...nicely! Hopefully this means Andrew is on the mend. He had thirteen hours sleep last night and his antibiotics are finished.

Tuesday, 16th December 2014
Andrew was nil-by-mouth at the Royal Marsden for his lumbar puncture this morning, but we were sent home as his chest was too congested and the anaesthetist was not inclined to 'put him under'. They are going to ring me with a rescheduled date before Christmas.

Wednesday, 17th December 2014
Andrew is asleep; Clara is at a play date. I am relaxing drinking Baileys whilst watching a film with my husband. Purely medicinal.

Scrap that moment. Andrew has woken up with a temperature of 39.9, so we are off to get him checked out at the Queen Elizabeth.

Thursday, 18th December 2014

Neutrophils 0.4. CRP 80, which might indicate a bacterial infection and would require five days of IV antibiotics, depending on the results of the blood cultures, so maybe we will be out on the evening of 23rd. His white blood count is a little low, but otherwise his blood picture is looking very good (not a relapse). Andrew's been checked over three times: by the junior doctor, then the senior doctor, and finally the registrar. The registrar thinks one lung is sounding a little different from the other and suspects the bacteria are in there. An X-ray will tell us more. Andrew is still spiking high temperatures, so he is having regular Calpol. The IV antibiotics have been started. Goodness knows what is going on. It is my work Christmas do tonight, with a bit of jazz, in Streatham. I am going to go, but I am trying not to feel too guilty about being out when Joseph and Andrew are in hospital and Clara is at Grandma's house.

Friday, 19th December 2014

Andrew's CRP is higher, at 132, and we are waiting for the blood cultures, which will be back at 7pm. The CRP lags behind infection, so is high even if he is feeling better. We had a visit from the Woolwich Barracks Soldiers and "that wasn't the real" Father Christmas with three presents, which cheered us all up, especially the very silly turkey hat.

Saturday, 20th December 2014

The results today from the blood cultures and throat swab are both negative, but the CRP is still high, at 58, and Andrew is still neutropenic. We are planning on another night in hospital. He will be having IV antibiotics. Hopefully we can come home tomorrow morning with oral antibiotics, if all is still well and if the CRP comes down. This is not exactly how I wanted to spend the last weekend before Christmas. Clara is here to keep us occupied. Joseph has gone for two more concerts at the Royal Albert Hall. Was that only a week ago?!

Sunday, 21st December 2014

Joseph gets a boy in hospital who sleeps until 8am or 9am; this morning I get a boy who pings awake at 6am and is then given a dose of antibiotics, which keep failing, as his Wiggly keeps occluding, and the only way to make it work is for him to sit up with his hand on his head! "I'm hungry!" "I need a wee!" I think someone may be better. Oh, and no cough yet!

This afternoon we are Ho… Ho… Home! Neutrophils are only 0.1, so we are on lockdown until the big day.

Monday, 22nd December 2014

Andrew has spent the happiest hour opening all his cards from friends at school. He was thrilled with each and every one. I am also overwhelmed that, in the little time he has been at school, he has made a felt stocking and a Christmas card for us. His class even made a 'Get Well Soon' book and each child wrote a message and drew a picture. He loves it so much and wanted me to read it as his bedtime story tonight. Brilliant, Balgowan Primary School.

A doctor at the Royal Marsden made my day by postponing Andrew's lumbar puncture, due tomorrow, until the New Year. "Wouldn't want to make him ill again". Yippee!

Wednesday, 24th December 2014
We are 8 grandchildren, 6 parents, 2 grandparents, 1 dog and a high tide in St Osyth. Let the fun and festivities begin!

Thursday, 25th December 2014
Merry Christmas, everybody. I am hoping you and yours are happy and healthy. We had a lie in until 7am - score! We are off now for a lovely walk to a bird hide in the Essex countryside.

Friday 26th December 2014
I am in bed with my Andrew Bear who is building 'Star Wars' Lego. Someone else is cooking a fry up. Clara is dancing around listening to her new (my old) iPod shuffle with all of Caroline and Pasha's 'Strictly Come Dancing' songs on it. Love it.

Monday, 29th December 2014
We are home. The children are asleep. Joseph is out. I am in my pyjamas, ready to start a Christmas TV marathon as I have watched nothing at all so far. Up first it has to be 'Miranda'.

Tuesday, 30th December 2014
Bloods have been done at home this morning. Let's hope for some neutrophils. Andrew *really* wants to go to the cinema to see 'Penguins of Madagascar'!

Wednesday, 31st December 2014

This year Andrew has:

Taken approximately two thousand two hundred and thirty tablets of chemotherapy and antibiotics,

Had ten weeks with no immune system,

Spent thirteen nights in hospital with sixty lots of IV antibiotics,

Visited the Royal Marsden four times for IV vincristine chemo,

Visited another four times for lumbar punctures.

Visited the Queen Elizabeth for eight lots of IV vincristine chemo injections,

Had three physio appointments,

Given seven urine samples,

Had six chest x-rays,

Had one throat swab,

Had two tests for chickenpox,

Had three nose swabs,

Had twelve weeks of steroids,

Had forty visits from the local nurses to have bloods taken at home,

Missed around six weeks of school.

Taken part in the Race for Life,

And organised a Santa Fun Run.

We have:

Raised one thousand two hundred and ninety eight pounds for cancer charities,

Shot each other with lasers in the woods, thanks to the Emily Ash Trust,

Had a fabulous weekend in Centre Parcs, thanks to Lucy's Day Out,

And received new bikes from Cyclists Fighting Cancer.

This is our third New Year with cancer. We have taken a big step forward towards the end of treatment. This time next year, (hopefully), we may be eight weeks off finishing. I am so proud of Andrew, of Clara, of all the Berthouds. Happy New Year, one and all, family, old friends and new. Thank you for keeping me going and enjoy every minute of 2015.

Friday, 2nd January 2015

A fellow cancer mummy arrived at our local hospital last night, with a poorly child, to discover no TVs were working in any of the four rooms or in the communal area. An email to Chartwell Cancer Trust (who approved money) and a quick dash to Curry's later, I arrived at the Queen Elizabeth with new remotes, batteries and aerials. The parents set to work and now all the TVs work! I feel like I did a good deed indeed, but what makes me feel cross is the fact that all four rooms were occupied over Christmas with no TVs working and, of course, no Wi-Fi. Try forty-eight hours in hospital with a child and no TV or Wi-Fi! Huge thanks to the Chartwell Cancer Trust for being so supportive.

Sunday, 4th January 2015

The very beautiful Mia was in the Royal Marsden and diagnosed with leukaemia at the same time as us. I remember her watching EastEnders and I remember her lovely long plaits. I also remember thinking how hard it must be for her, being diagnosed in Year Six, and how fortunate we were that Andrew was only three years old. But today she has completed her cancer journey and, how utterly fabulous that today is her last day of chemotherapy! She is at the end of her treatment and I am so pleased for her and her family.

Friday, 9th January 2015

Oh, the joy of a day off and one which involves me, shops, coffee and no hospitals, work or poorly small people.

Wednesday, 14th January 2015

I am so stupid, as Andrew is due a lumbar puncture on Friday for intrathecal (IT) methotrexate chemo, but I gave him his weekly dose of oral methotrexate tonight and he can't have both (again – I have done this before). We, therefore, have to get the lumbar puncture postponed. Last night I forgot to give him the mercaptopurine chemo at all. I am too tired to function at the moment.

Friday, 23rd January 2015

I am enjoying some quality time with Andrew on my day off whilst we wait for his lumbar puncture under general anaesthetic at the Royal Marsden.

Sunday, 25th January 2015

My Bromley Childhood Cancer Support Group are meeting up this morning. The children are giggling and munching popcorn whilst watching 'Penguins of Madagascar'. Two new families have joined us this month. Thanks to the Beckenham Odeon for a private screening, which enables even neutropenic children to come with no risk of infection.

Happy children, happy parents, happy times.

Wednesday, 28 January 2015

Andrew is on the way back from hospital. He was sick several times in the night and had a high temperature, so we popped in this morning for him to be checked over.

Fortunately, he has 5 whole neutrophils (that is high!) so he can come home and recover like a normal poorly five-year-old.

Friday, 20th January 2015

Not quite the day off I had planned, as I now have Andrew in tow. My massage was scrapped, but Andrew enjoyed chocolate cake, biscuits, apple juice and a 'Star Wars' magazine whilst I had my haircut. We have since safely arrived at a hotel in Southampton for a weekend of relaxation and time with the Cross family. Clara is impressed already with the 'posh' toilets and 'pink moisturiser that smells mmmmm.' Andrew is amazed we have a bath AND a shower, and me? There is an espresso coffee machine in the room!

Friday, 6th February 2015

I have had a fun Friday: first, a free Caffe Nero coffee, followed by a much-needed massage; then I managed to send my NPQH (headship course) application form off before 1pm. Yippee! Now however I am confused. Whoo, Whoo, red alert! Red alert! It is steroid week and Andrew DOES NOT want pizza!

Saturday 7th February 2015

Phew. Pizza panic over. Normality resumed. We are having lunch at Pizza Express.

Wednesday, 11th February 2015

Two exasperations of the day:
1. Turns out it might be a dodgy batch of steroids which caused Andrew's recent sickness/upset tummy.

2. Three new children have been diagnosed with cancer in Bromley recently.

Saturday, 14th February 2015

We are nice and cosy in the Emily Ash Trust caravan, having another much-needed respite break. We are very grateful to be back for some family time in Battle near Hastings.

Sunday, 15th February 2015

Today we have enjoyed two hours swimming in the caravan park's pool and then four hours at Bodiam Castle. I am ready for a nap!

Monday, 16th February 2015

Oh, we do like to be beside the sea side; oh, we do like to be beside the sea! Today we have enjoyed fish and chips, crazy golf, arcades, rides, ice creams and the beach at Hastings seafront and a walk along the Promenade.

Tuesday, 17th February 2015

We had a 'bloods party' today when Emma and Ollie came to the Crowhurst caravan and the Hastings community nurses came to us and did both blood tests. Emma and Ollie were diagnosed a few days before us and we met them in the Royal Marsden.

Friday, 20th February 2015

When we were told Andrew had cancer we were advised the treatment would be three years long, as he was a boy. Treatment length is different because research showed, if boys stop treatment at two years, like girls, it is more likely their disease will return (a relapse). What they didn't say was it was three years from the beginning of the intensive chemotherapy phase called Escalating Capizzi. We started this on February 20th 2013, four and a half months after diagnosis. Today is February 20th 2015. If Andrew was a girl, he would be taking his last ever chemotherapy tonight; he would have had his last ever steroids and last ever lumbar puncture. But blood cancer can hide in testicles and so we must do another year to prevent a relapse.

We are on the final countdown:

Three hundred and sixty-five days of mercaptopurine chemo to go,
Twelve steroids weeks,
Four lumbar punctures,
Fifty-six more times accessing Andrew's port for bloods and chemotherapy.

We have completed two years four months and three weeks of treatment, something which seemed impossible once; one more year will fly by!

Friday, 27th February 2015
The sun is shining and Andrew has been to school. Some of his classmates were awarded one hundred percent attendance certificates today. We're celebrating Andrew's first full week at school since November instead.

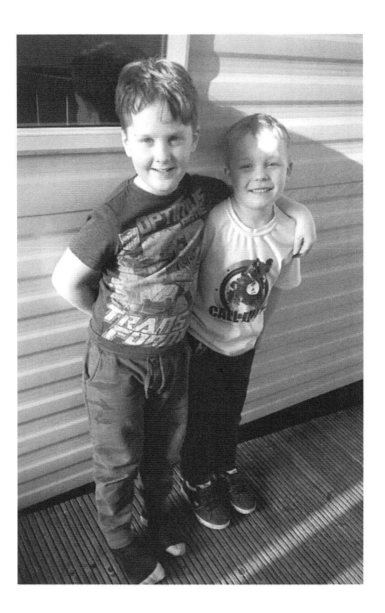

Chapter 15

Long Term Maintenance – Cycle 8

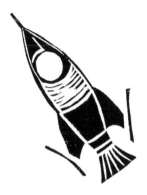

Cancer takes you hostage

Pain, dark, lonely then it is

Lightness, over? Free?

Monday, 2nd March 2015

Cycle Eight of Maintenance started today with IV vincristine chemotherapy at the Royal Marsden. Joseph collected another two hundred beads of courage. Steroid week has started so Andrew is being a MasterChef and making homemade pizza.

Wednesday, 4th March 2015

I am heartbroken. It has taken me twenty-five minutes to persuade Andrew to leave the house. "I feel like my brain has gone. I wish I didn't have leukaemia. I don't like this." Blooming steroids. A bit of chocolate in the glove box of the car got him up and out of the house in the end.

We attended Clara's concert at school this afternoon so his teacher sent Andrew home with us at 3pm rather than 3:30pm. He was sleepy but still managed his day. We are so grateful to the school for keeping him going. Day Three done!

Thursday, 5th March 2015

Andrew was downhearted and sleepy at 9am again today - Joseph brought him back home where he promptly slept for two hours. He woke up bonny and bouncy, so did the rest of the day at school. He's like an eighteen-month-old: up at 6am and back to sleep at 9am.

Wednesday, 11th March 2015

I am donating £3 to Macmillan, not to say #sozmum but #thanksmum. We are having new windows installed in our house, so we have moved in with Mum and Dad for a week (or so). It is heavenly to have a dust- and mess-free haven to escape to after a busy day at work, plus all the extra help with feeding and childcare.

Thursday, 12th March 2015

CCLASP - http://cclasp.co.uk/ - you have made our month with your enormous bag of goodies for Andrew. Your generosity towards us, after a difficult steroid week, is wonderful and very gratefully received.

Sunday, 15th March 2015

I have had a perfect mother's day. Joseph and the children were away overnight so I woke up at 9am, made myself breakfast in bed and watched a film. The family returned for lunch with cards and flowers. I had a cuddle with my mum and then an afternoon of fun, Prosecco and dinner with the Perrotts.

Tuesday, 17th March 2015

Andrew is back, awake and eating after his lumbar Puncture at the Royal Marsden. Our consultant is still very pleased with his progress and he is still in remission and cancer-free.

Friday, 20th March 2015

We are at the Queen Elizabeth, having Andrew's chickenpox immunity tested, as one of Andrew's friends has come out in spots today.

Saturday, 21st March 2015

Yes! Andrew still has immunity to chickenpox. Exhale. No nasty ZIG jab needed here, but boo - Clara has tonsillitis.

Sunday 22ⁿᵈ March 2015

Not quite the Sunday we had planned. Clara's tonsillitis means she's had high temperatures, so although we have booked and fundraised we have decided the Royal Marsden Sponsored walk (or Marsden March) is not possible this year. We are currently snuggled up under a duvet, watching 'Matilda' and eating hot cross buns. Sorry to those who sponsored us, but your money is still going to the most amazing hospital, where the facilities, doctors and nurses make paediatric oncology much more bearable.

Wednesday, 25ᵗʰ March 2015

It is 00:02 so I can say Happy Birthday to Joseph who is whizzing to hospital with Andrew because he woke up burning hot, being sick and with a headache. Not quite the birthday breakfast I had planned. Clara is going to be devastated to find no Andrew or Daddy at home in the morning. Now to try to calm my adrenaline enough to go back to sleep.

An evening update: Andrew has had high temperatures on and off all day; the highest was 39.4; they recorded 38.3 just now, so it is creeping up again. He is not managing to keep down the oral paracetamol, so we resorted to giving it via IV in the end; plus, he is having a slow drip feed bag of fluids to rehydrate him after all the sickness. Joseph is home with Clara so I am snuggled up in hospital. We managed a brief present opening and singing of Happy Birthday here in the hospital after school. Thanks for all your well wishes and messages - they made Andrew very smiley tonight. Clara finds the disruption and forced separation very hard so some TLC in her direction, if you see her, would be great too.

Thursday, 26th March 2015

At 5pm the doctors took Andrew's fluids down. No medicine was needed until midday tomorrow, so I asked what the benefit was of staying at hospital versus going home. They couldn't think of any, sooooo we're HOME!

Friday, 27th March 2015

Andrew had his midday antibiotics and is allowed home until the same time tomorrow. We picked up eighty-five Easter eggs from Virgin Money in Bromley. The fundraising manager read about my support group in the Chartwell Cancer Trust magazine and contacted head office to see if they could collect Easter eggs for us. Their customers have been donating them into the store. How wonderful!

Saturday, 28th March 2015

It's midday and we are back at the Queen Elizabeth for antibiotics and to be checked over again by Dr Schuller. Andrew has had two mild migraines since we were here yesterday. However, there have been no big concerns; he still has a viral infection, so we are home, de-accessed, and with no need to go back again before vincristine and steroids on Tuesday.

Sunday, 29th March 2015

We had a fun-tastic Easter Party for Bromley oncology children and their siblings in Knockholt. Mr. Marvel – the children's entertainer - held everyone's attention. Huge thanks to the Mr. Marvel Company for waiving their admin fee. Three of the oncology siblings bonded and had a fabulous time doing an Easter egg hunt. That makes me so satisfied and is totally the point of the group.

Monday, 30th March 2015
I have made Andrew a steroid countdown rocket, which is up and ready to be coloured in, starting tomorrow with Day One of sixty left. We all need to see that the number of steroid days we have to cope with are diminishing.

Friday, 31st March 2015
Goodness. I spoke to the man who rented out the village hall and he's reimbursed the deposit AND the hire charge for Sunday's oncology Easter party. He was totally taken with the children, the group and the photos. He said we can contact anytime to try and use it AND someone in the village rents out a bouncy castle! People are so lovely.

Saturday, 1st April 2015
The oncology ward at the Queen Elizabeth have been wanting their own kitchen for families. Small pleasures, like making a cup of tea or making a meal for grownups, have been impossible. In December 2014, Michael Douglas (from CCT) visited Tiger Ward at the Queen Elizabeth Hospital and met with the Macmillan paediatric nurse. He promised to help turn the bathroom into a kitchen by pledging the five thousand pounds to make it happen.

Today it opened after a very speedy process. We celebrated with a party today (everyone got an Easter egg) and Michael cut the ribbon. The staff at the Queen Elizabeth have always been fantastic, and now they have a provision to match them. This is the continuation of a beautiful relationship between CCT and the Bromley oncology children. Chartwell Cancer Trust have now set up a new branch of the charity for us called CCT Tiger Ward: http://chartwellcancertrust.co.uk/tiger-ward/ . In the near future, a new full-time health care assistant will be funded by CCT and Michael wants the facilities at Tiger Ward to rival those of Great Ormond Street Hospital.

Tuesday, 7th April 2015

I have been totally floored by either a migraine, which lasted twenty-four hours, or possibly sinusitis. Either way I have spent the last two days in bed and only now feel well enough to sit up and open the curtain. On the plus side, Joseph is now going to enforce mummy duvet days, so I don't exhaust myself again. Work, going into hospital, having the children at home for Easter, and Andrew on steroids, has wiped me out.

Thursday, 16th April 2015

I have just watched the BBC documentary 'Raining in my Heart' from last night. Every word is true. Children with cancer are braver than they know and stronger than adults. They know no different so accept it all with grace and a smile. Those parents said everything I and every cancer parent has ever thought. Every day is special. We want them to live the best life they can. There is no choice other than to fill our children will poison and high toxicity to kill the cancer and hopefully not kill them.

"It is like being on a rocket to the moon- you cannot get off."

I love that quote - one day you're walking along in life and suddenly you get dragged onto a rocket with no warning and no chance to pause, pack, prepare or think for even a second. It was an utterly wonderful documentary but totally devastating too because of the reality of those children whose journey has ended with an explosion of love and bravery. These children are in the sky, in the stars, twinkling forever above us.

For us, the rocket has been flying for two and a half years and I hope we continue to be one of the lucky ones and land our rocket safely back on the ground

Friday, 24th April 2015
Pretty perfect day off. I had a massage, a haircut, a cheese and wine lunch with Joseph followed by a two hour nap. The children are on play-dates after school, so that we can enjoy mojitos and mezze in South Kensington with my father-in-law, Richard. Now we have free tickets to see Richard sing at the Royal Albert Hall!

Sunday, 26th April 2015
We had a superb complimentary party for the BCCSG cancer meet up this morning at Pizza Express, Beckenham. It was lovely to see the oncology family. All the children made their own pizzas and the staff played games with them whilst they cooked.

Thursday, 30th April 2015
Andrew woke me at 5:30am wanting to burrow into bed with me (Day Four of steroids) and he promptly fell back to sleep. I was feeling a bit miffed, as I was wide awake, but then this photo of a bald, skinny cancer kid popped up on my Facebook feed, so I can't take my eyes off him. I love him to bits.

Tuesday, 5th May 2015

Since getting home from work I have been:

Painting a Death Star piñata (was a football),

Freezing Han in Carbonite (coloured ice),

Laminating 'Pin the Light Sabre on Yoda,'

Baking Chewbacca biscuits,

Blowing up stormtrooper skittles,

Creating 'Knock Down the AT AT' out of photocopier boxes,

Writing out instructions for 'Don't Drop Yoda',

Blowing up green glowstick light sabres,

And printing and laminating Chewbacca, Yoda and stormtrooper masks!

Next Year when Andrew wants a football party I will let him!

Wednesday, 6th May 2015

We are totally shattered after two hours with Andrew's class for a Star Wars party. Never again! "You're a great party girl, Mummy," he said. So it was all worthwhile. Good job he's super special and I love him.

Wednesday, 13th May 2015

No chemotherapy! It has been a long time since we had a break in daily oral mercaptopurine chemo. During 'hair falling out/throwing up daily' chemotherapy, we looked forward to the rest weeks, but now, on Maintenance, we have more or less given Andrew mercaptopurine every day at bedtime for two years. Anyway his immune system is compromised today: neutrophils are only 0.3. So no chemotherapy for a week to let them recover and extra hand-washing is needed. We have a week of pretending there is no cancer and more time for Pimms in the sunshine.

Monday, 18th May 2015

I am nervous but excited. I phoned Starlight Children's Foundation today to get the ball rolling with Andrew's end of treatment wish. Nine months to go! http://www.starlight.org.uk/

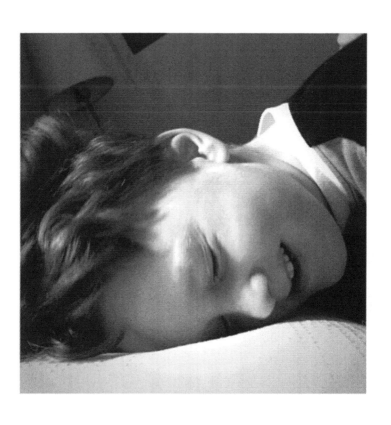

Chapter 16

Long Term Maintenance – Cycle 9

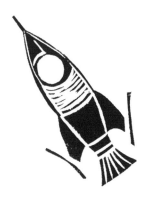

Try to be normal

But what does normal mean now?

How can we forget?

Tuesday, 26th May 2015

I am so thankful to the doctors and nurses at the Royal Marsden Hospital. Another twelve weeks completed and another step closer to the end of treatment. Cycle Nine of twelve started. Andrew is still cancer-free and in remission.

Thursday, 28th May 2015

We are at Coolings Nature Trail for a nice short walk. It is Day Three of steroids. There are lots of new things to look at here, including the 'tree of memories'. This is a tree in the middle of the grounds where visitors can tie their wristbands to the branches to remember a loved one. Donations from the tree will go to the Chartwell Cancer Trust. Andrew and Clara, of course, wanted to donate some money for 'us'.

Sunday, 31st May 2015

Fabulous day! Many thanks to the Emily Ash Trust and Country Wide Special Events for another fun-filled family day. You saw how much the oncology kids and siblings appreciated all your efforts. For us parents, it is another day of fun, laughter and memories to be cherished. We loved running around in the woods dressed as soldiers shooting each other with laser guns!

Saturday, 6th June 2015

We have had a super special family day out in Ware, Hertford, with all the Berthouds, for my nephew William's christening. I am three times a godmother now.

Monday, 8th June 2015

Andrew: "Mummy, tomorrow I want two boxes of Coco Pops, apple juice and a ham sandwich." Love him. This means only one thing. It is nil-by-mouth lumbar puncture day at the Royal Marsden. Andrew requests his food before he is anaesthetised. Knowing what he is going to eat afterwards somehow enables him to cope with not eating for hours.

Tuesday, 9th June 2015
Andrew's coughing a lot, (the typical croupy cough he seems to get), so I was not sure if they would do the general anaesthetic today, but I took him in anyway.

His chest was clear so the doctor was happy. The anaesthetist was also willing to go ahead. They didn't intubate him (put a tube down his throat), but used a mask over his mouth instead. Not being able to have a drink made the dry tickly cough worse.

The 'Despicable Me 2' party scene was put on the TV, for him to watch for thirty seconds while he was being put under. I made a quick run to the cafe for breakfast and coffee before he came back out.

You know the scene in 'Big Hero 6' where Baymax is running out of battery and falling over everywhere as if he's drunk? That was Andrew, eating his Coco Pops.

Friday, 12th June 2015
I disappeared into an Ofsted fog on Wednesday, just as Andrew was spiking temperatures, 0.1 degree off having to be admitted. Well done, Super Daddy and Mum for holding the fort at home. It was lovely to see the mini Berthouds finally tonight (after not seeing them since Wednesday morning).

Monday, 22nd June 2015

I can't sleep. My head is buzzing with work and the anxiety of steroid week beginning tomorrow. After this week there are only seven to go, which is NOTHING! So I am actually a bit excited too. Be still, brain.

Monday, 29th June 2015

A month ago my nephew began, what we now know to be, his cancer journey. Not leukaemia, this time, but a rhabdomyosarcoma in his testicle. Friday gave them the best possible news: that no other tumours were found, and so his twenty-two weeks of chemotherapy can begin today at Great Ormond Street Hospital. Having a child with cancer is utterly devastating. Having two young cousins, both three years and five months at diagnosis, has rocked our world. I remember being told he had gone into hospital with a lump and I felt like the ground under me was lurching with shock. We couldn't say so at the time, but Clara wrote on her Race for Life bib that she was running for both Andrew and her cousin, (little) Joseph. So thank you for all the sponsorship, as she raised over three hundred pounds.

Cancer, leave our children alone.

Thursday, 2nd July

When Andrew was first diagnosed, I couldn't think about anything other than cancer. Socialising with others was incredibly hard as other people's frippery was so meaningless compared to the everyday trials and tribulations of a child undergoing treatment.

Somehow, without my knowing it, that has changed. Tonight I enjoyed a great night out with class mums, listening to the stories of others and I realised, as I have come to realise more and more, that everyone has a life story to share. Everyone has heartache in their lives, and love and joy, but not everyone chooses to share it.

Today Andrew had his 'meet the new teacher' day. When he was diagnosed with cancer at three years and five months, we were told the treatment would be three years long and I remember thinking: he will be in Year Two when he finishes. That seemed unimaginable - an eon away. Yet suddenly he has met his Year Two teachers today and it all seems suddenly close and very real.

One day we won't be living with this nightmare anymore and it will become another story we choose to share (or not) with others. Thank you for reading and sharing our journey. Thank you for giving us space to be 'fine' when we're not and for listening when we're ready to talk. But most of all, thanks for the great nights out which make me feel 'normal' again.

Monday, 8th July 2015
Four more working days until the summer holidays. Woohoo! Nearly the end of term.

Four days before the summer holidays end I'll be saying woohoo to sending the children back to school too, but for now I am looking forward to weeks of family time, festivals, camping, cuddles and fun (and two more steroid weeks ticked off) with the mini Berthouds.

Tuesday, 14th July 2015

I feel like a fairy godmother tonight, as I am putting money into the accounts of the oncology families. A huge thank you to the Chartwell Cancer Trust for allowing BCCSG families to have a fun filled family day out over the summer break.

Wednesday, 15th July 2015

Last day of work for forty-eight days!

Friday, 17th July 2015

For the next six weeks…

I will be a mum, not a working mum.
I will read books, not emails.
I will look at my children, not my phone/laptop.
I will see and talk to my friends more than work colleagues.
I will have 'meetings' which stretch on all day with my children, to listen to them and their ideas.
I will 'train' them to develop and grow into the best they can be.
And I will try to enjoy every argument and frustrating moment because in six weeks' time
I will miss them like mad.

Monday, 20th July 2015

Andrew and I are at Pizza Express, in Blackheath. We arrived at the hospital for this month's vincristine and dexamethasone, but for some reason, the vincristine hadn't been made up, so we had to go away and have lunch. One dose of steroids, so where else would we be but Pizza Express?

Thursday, 23rd July 2015

Day Four of steroids. We have survived in a flurry of IKEA meatballs, naps, the local park, noodles and 'Spy Kids 2'. Andrew has been very hungry, bored, grumpy and clingy. A new hurdle this month has been Andrew being bored of all the foods he 'has had in his life.' He wants something new, though getting a steroid child to try anything new is impossible. So it has been a Catch 22 situation, which he wants to fix by eating Coco Pops or cake, whereas I want him to eat carrot sticks or tomatoes.

He has also needed lots of cuddles and affection and if I have been unable to do this, (due to needing both hands for a task), he has been placated by standing RIGHT next to me or stroking my arm. Sometimes he creeps up behind me and I bonk him on the head with my elbow accidently. He even wanted me not to drive the car or to swap sides in the car so he could hold hands with me. At about 6pm he settled with a big box of Lego for about five minutes whilst Clara was amusing herself (and not vying for my attention, in direct competition with Andrew) and I let out a relaxed sigh.

Foolish, as the five minutes ended and Andrew was next to me, fiddling with Clara's Chop Stix, and managed, somehow, to snap them in two. Chop-Stix-Gate almost started world war three. Clara was furious; Andrew was devastated and dejected. She ranted. He stormed off to hide in bed, as did I with a book. Day Five tomorrow - almost done for another month.

Monday, 27th July 2015

We celebrated our 13th wedding anniversary with a marvellous day in Swanage. We took a ride on the steam train, completed the kids' trail around Corfe castle, and followed it with rides at the seafront funfair. The children swam in the sea and made sand castles on the beach. We finished with a delicious country pub dinner.

Tuesday, 28th July 2015

For the last one hundred and forty-seven weeks we have had weekly blood tests - Andrew's port is accessed to withdraw blood to be tested in the lab. Last year, when we were in Swanage, we drove around to Poole Hospital to have Andrew's bloods done. When in Hastings, the community nurses come to us, but this week we have been allowed to have a week off! Last week was steroid week, which usually causes Andrew's blood levels to be high. So this week, there will be no accessing, no blood results, no using up a day's holiday. Very exciting!

Saturday, 1st August 2015

It is startling to think of the number of places in which we have given Andrew his daily chemotherapy. When Andrew was diagnosed with cancer I thought chemotherapy meant sitting in a hospital with a drip attached to his arm, like Walter White in 'Breaking Bad'. Little did I know chemotherapy was 'medicine', which came in tablet-form and could be given anywhere. We gave Andrew his daily mercaptopurine chemo tonight in our tent at Camp Bestival. It got me to thinking of all the places outside of hospital we have given Andrew chemotherapy over the last few years:

Granny's house in St. Osyth
Grandma's house in Beckenham
Holiday house in Bungay, Suffolk
Travelodge in Windsor
Legoland Hotel
Hotel in Margate
Hotel in Towersey
Holiday House in Swanage
'Telfordfest' camp site
'Berthoud fest' barn in Telford
Camp site in Epping, Essex
Hotel in Southampton
Andy and Polly's house in Southampton
Crowhurst Park in Battle
Centre Parcs Lodge in Norfolk

The only problem, on a camp site, is keeping the chemotherapy somewhere secure and safe. If the car is nearby, then we can keep it in the lockable glove box; if not then we keep it in my lockable suitcase.

Monday, 3rd August 2015
We are home from the festival with filthy children, dirty clothes, no voices (I have got laryngitis), and split heels, feeling totally shattered. The carpet feels oddly soft; the toilet is not smelly, and it is so nice to sit in an armchair. Thank you, Camp Bestival, you were A-MAZING!

Thursday, 13th August 2015
Summers in the UK probably don't get much better than a day on Southwold beach with new wetsuits and body-boards. Happy children. Happy Mummy. I am so blessed to have my family around me.

Monday, 17ᵗʰ August 2015

On the eve of the start of Andrew's penultimate cycle of chemotherapy, I am overwhelmed at how far we have come. From a scrummy toddler to a handsome boy, via 'the cancer years'. For those of you at the start of your journey, (and especially with boys), the end of treatment seems like a lifetime away. It feels like it most of the time, but then suddenly it is racing towards you. Another day done everyone.

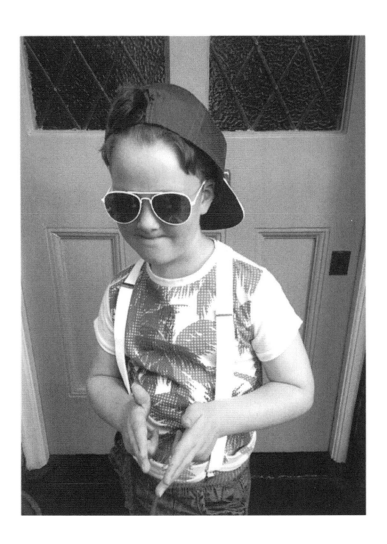

Chapter 17

Long Term Maintenance – Cycle 10

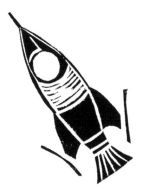

The light at the end

Of the tunnel is getting

Closer day by day

Tuesday, 18th August 2015

We saw our consultant today. Andrew is still cancer-free and in remission. Maintenance Cycle Ten of twelve - the next twelve-week cycle has begun with steroids and IV vincristine chemo. Sending love and hugs to Andrew's cousin, Joseph, who was having vincristine at the same time in a different hospital - brave boys. Super Andrew was then whizzed back to Purley, Croydon for 'music week', as he didn't want to miss his ukulele lesson! Love him.

Thursday, 20th August 2015

Six months of daily chemotherapy left until 20th February 2016. The light at the end of the tunnel is getting closer.

I am managing 'Andrew's steroids vs Music Week' by collecting him at lunchtime and taking him for a drive around the block. Hopefully a thirty minute snooze will be enough to get him through ukuleles, a talent show and a party this afternoon. Day Three of steroids.

Friday, 21st August 2015

Day Four of steroids and Mr. Awesome Andrew managed his music week concert (after a two-hour nap), singing, playing the recorder and the ukulele. Special mention to Clara who was a confident cookie throughout, also singing, playing the ukulele and leading a group with her recorder. We are celebrating by going out for dinner.

Sunday, 23rd August 2015

The cancer countdown rocket is half full: a hundred and sixty-eight nights of oral chemotherapy, two lumbar punctures, six injections of vincristine and only six pulses of dreaded steroids left.

Monday, 24th August 2015

I have spoken to Andrew's wish-maker at Starlight Children's Foundation. She is in the process of sorting out his wish for the end of his treatment. He wants to 'fly to Greece and snorkel in the sea'. Our consultant has given the go ahead for him to fly, so now we are on to the next stage of preparations.

Tuesday, 25th August 2015

Having a 'happy memory making' day at Chessington World of Adventures, all thanks to a charity called Forward Facing: http://www.forwardfacing.co.uk/ It has been so lovely to spend the day with my oncology family too. It was so fabulous to talk; you keep me sane AND, as a few rides were shut, we all get to come back another day completely free!

P.S. I feel sick after being made to go on Vampire and Dragon's Fury.

Wednesday, 26th August 2015

It feels wonderful when members of the oncology family reach the end of their treatment. Erin wasn't diagnosed until almost a year after us but has had the go ahead to end all chemotherapy today - girls with leukaemia complete one year less than boys. Now the road to recovery begins for you, Erin, and I wish you all the happiness in the world. Still we plod on to our End of Treatment on 20th February 2016.

Saturday, 29th August 2015

We had an exciting afternoon at Apollo Victoria Theatre for our family day out, paid for by the Chartwell Cancer Trust.

I was an emotional wreck after the 'for good' finale. Then Glinda made an announcement about a previous cast member who has a relapsed cancer and needs sending out of the UK for treatment. Could we donate money to the cause via cast members holding buckets? Yes! So on the way out the children met one of the flying monkeys who was holding a bucket for donations.

Sunday, 30th August 2015

I hosted a lovely BCCSG meet up this morning at Coolings Nature Trail. We arrived before hours to 'wake up' the animals and give them their breakfast: a special experience behind the scenes, with lots of fascinating information from the Head Ranger, followed, of course, with delicious tea and cake or hot chocolate and bacon sandwiches. Thank you to Chartwell Cancer Trust for the suggestion. Now we are off to Towersey Folk Festival!

Monday, 31st August 2015

We have one last day at the festival before going home to start back at work and school. As the moral of the Disney Film, 'Inside Out', goes - you need to experience sadness to understand happiness and vice versa; they go hand in hand. As a family, we have had an abundance of happy times this summer, thanks to a lot of wonderful people. Our happiness overfloweth. Hopefully our bank will be fully charged now, to get us through one last winter on treatment, and will not be too depleted by infections and hospital stays.

Thursday, 3rd September 2015

I shall be posting first day of school photos on Monday, not today. The happiness cup has been slightly depleted overnight. Andrew moaned and groaned all night long and then was finally sick at 6am. How utterly frustrating.

Monday, 7th September 2015
Finally, both children are back at school and hopefully this is the year Andrew finishes treatment for cancer. I met his new teachers last week, on their INSET day, and was able to explain his treatment in detail up until February.

After that, we will have to wait and see. I emailed the new headteacher and explained Andrew's situation, but he already knew and has agreed to the children having time off for Disneyland Paris in March and our BIG wish holiday next June.

Tuesday, 8th September 2015
Some of Andrew's original symptoms, in the run up to being diagnosed with leukaemia, were lethargy, nose bleeds and being sick. So this past week, after three nose bleeds, three times being sick and very tired on different days, I have been in an internal panic. Relapse means, quite literally, a 'recurrence of the past,' and I have been scared, except for the fact that his bloods have been perfectly normal. Having a blood cancer means surely something would show up in his weekly blood test?

So I was keeping everything crossed for today's blood results, which were phoned in promptly three hours after being taken and were all perfectly healthy and normal. He has plenty of platelets, a normal number of white blood cells and high neutrophils. I am sure all the dancing at the folk festival may have been a step too far and he was exhausted with a cold which might have led to his symptoms. It goes to show how, nearing the end of treatment, your mind plays tricks on you and you don't quite believe that one day this might actually be over.

Thursday, 10th September 2015
Andrew's having a lumbar puncture at the Royal Marsden today with Daddy whilst I go to work. I am looking forward to threading on the next lot of beads of courage tonight.

Monday, 14th September 2015
All Year One and Two children are now having the flu nasal spray as part of their childhood immunisations - great! Except the live vaccine is dangerous for Andrew. I now need to book him in for a flu jab, as soon as possible, and before his peers at school have the nasal spray. I have rung my GP, to book an appointment for the week after next, as Andrew cannot have the jab whilst on steroids. However, I have been told I cannot book an appointment with them until I have been invited to book an appointment by them in a letter, which they are posting to me this week. Silent scream. This is like the 'your son is obese, please ring us urgently' reception weight check all over again.

Tuesday, 15th September 2015
Since the beginning of term, Clara has been driven by the desire to bake cakes with her friends and sell them after school as a fundraiser for a cancer charity. I finally relented and let the three of them do it today. The bake-off resulted in lots of yummy cakes for neighbours and passers-by with a total of £42.25 raised! I am very proud of her - just don't look at my kitchen!

Thursday, 17th September 2015

When I was at our 'local' hospital, in Woolwich, on Tuesday, there was a new End of Treatment bell installed, the money for which had been raised entirely by another oncology child's sibling, the champion superstar, Ewan. We get to ring it three times and read out the poem:

> Ring this bell
> Three times well
> Its toll to clearly say
> My treatment's done
> The course is run
> And I am on my way

One girl has had this privilege, so far, since its recent installation - someone fully in remission from a Wilms' tumour. However, the scary, gut-wrenching part in the cycle of people ending their journey and ringing the bell, is the other children who start their rocket flight. Unfortunately, the Queen Elizabeth is full of newly diagnosed children, some with tumours, two within two hours of each other, and in the next six weeks, even more children will be diagnosed with cancer. Autumn is a peak time, for some awful reason. So thank you, Ewan for giving those children an end goal to aim for. How wonderfully resilient and motivated the older oncology siblings are.

Friday, 18th September 2015

Day Four of steroids. Andrew deserves a medal for surviving his first steroid week in Year Two. We will have to settle with a special 'bumpy' bead of courage instead. We were rung at lunchtime yesterday, as Andrew had taken himself to the medical room, feeling tired, but his lovely teacher talked to him and he decided to stay to design his Mexican mask. We've been so lucky with all of Andrew's teachers. The hard work they put into making school life fun, and worth staying for, means such a lot to us. Not only can we continue to work, but Andrew continues to socialise, maintain friendships and not have as many gaps in his learning as we feared he might. We had play-dates after school today and, after dinner, he stomped upstairs and put himself to bed. I just checked and Mr. Sleepy is fast asleep. One day left. Five pulses to go.

Thursday, 24th September 2015

OMG! I can't sit or stand still because of a phone call at 2:45pm from the Emily Ash Trust, asking me if I'd like to go tonight to see One Direction at the 02. The children are going to burst with excitement when I tell them.

Thank you - what a night! Clara turned to me and said, "Is this real or am I dreaming? I can't believe it!" The O2 was full of eighteen-year-old girls. I only knew three songs, but I loved every single minute. The look, all night, on Clara and Andrew's faces - big beaming grins, whilst jumping up and down waving light sticks - will stay with me forever. Magic. All for this Mrs. Amazing Cancer Sibling. I love you, Clara.

Saturday, 26th September 2015

Andrew's cancer diagnosis grounded us in the UK for the duration of his treatment (our choice on Maintenance), so Joseph has taken Clara to France for a weekend each year instead. This weekend it was Andrew's turn for a boy's overnight stay in Margate and a trip to Dreamland: six-year-old boy heaven. Great weather for it too! One of the rides was named after the signs of the zodiac, so Andrew chose the 'cancer' rocket. Andrew has a teddy monkey, Codling, whom he's had since birth, named after the midwife, Rebecca Codlin, so he was tickled pink to see a chippie sign selling codling and chips!

Sunday, 27th September 2015

I am currently sipping coffee whilst enjoying a private screening of Two by Two at the Beckenham Odeon this morning for the Bromley Childhood Cancer Support Group. It makes such a difference for children with suppressed immune systems to be able to go to the cinema without worrying about strange infections. All the children are munching popcorn and are happy!

Tuesday, 29th September 2015

This week I shall be distracting myself from the memories of three years ago, which led to us being told, on 3rd October 2012, that our three-year-old son had a life-threatening condition. Ever since that first day, I have kept a written and photo diary on Facebook of Andrew's experiences. At first it was a way of informing many people, as I only had to say something once when I couldn't face talking to anyone. After time though, people told me they were learning so much from my posts and I found it cathartic to write it all down, knowing that so many people were following and willing us along. I am looking forward to downloading all the posts and somehow getting them into a book for Andrew. I think I had better do it today after #facebookdown last night. It made me think I'd lose everything. How fantastic it will be when he is a teenager, or grown man, and he can read the diary of how wonderfully brave he was when he was aged three, four, five and six.

It constantly surprises me, throughout this journey, that people facing all sorts of cancers are drawing strength from us, adults included. A friend sent me this beautiful message:

"I want to thank you for the education and the inspiration. I know that what you have taught me helps me to understand the journeys of others and this makes me more use and support to them. I am proud to know you and honoured to watch this amazing example of motherhood, so thank you.

I started a cancer journey with my father a few months ago. In fact, I am with him today as he is having surgery and I feel that your posts have helped to prepare me for what will come: the daily stuff, the relentless issues and the length of time it will take. I know to pace myself. And I also know there will be joy and fun in there too. I hope I support him as well as you have Andrew. So simply, thanks".

Wednesday, 30 September 2015
Rest in Peace, a seventeen-year-old superstar whose rocket flight ended yesterday evening; he will forever be in the stars. No words can describe how we all feel. A small gesture, but I have donated money to the Teenage Cancer Trust (TCT) in your honour, as I know you worked hard to raise funds for them after your relapse. Be pain free and twinkle brightly.

Thursday, 1ˢᵗ October 2015
I would like to do one last Usborne order for the children at the Royal Marsden hospital. This will be the fourth and hopefully last Christmas Andrew will be on treatment.

Saturday, 3rd October 2015

I am spending our three year cancerversary away from the family, at a conference, in a hotel, with two hundred newly qualified teachers, which is a very useful distraction. Thank you for all your lovely time hop comments from 2012, 2013 and 2014. I have shed a tear reading through them all this morning. The pure shock expressed by your words, turning into pride for Andrew and us as a family is very emotional.

Joseph, Clara and Andrew are off to a special memory-making day at Zippo's Circus today. Fortunately, (unfortunately), they get to spend the day with their cousin who has also been invited to the 'Children with Cancer UK' special day: http://www.childrenwithcancer.org.uk/ Last night I raffled a class set of Lego, which I had been given, to the primary newly qualified teachers, and raised eighty-eight pounds for charity. Chartwell Cancer Trust, this will be coming your way. One thousand and ninety-five days of chemotherapy done; one hundred and thirty-five to go and counting.

The 2015 NQT residential conference for two hundred and twenty teachers is done and dusted. I have now collapsed on the sofa, looking at my beautiful 'thank you' flowers and awaiting the return of the mini Berthouds! Lucky me.

Monday, 5th October 2015

I hate having a poorly Clara – it always makes me feel scared and anxious. She was sent home from school and now has a temperature of 38.0.

Tuesday, 6th October 2015

Andrew's bloods have been taken for another week. Let's hope for some more neutrophils so we can get this flu jab done. He cannot have his flu jab on steroids or whilst neutropenic.

Thursday, 8th October 2015

The 'Kids Cancer Charity' have booked us three days and two nights at Disney's Newport Bay Club at Disneyland Paris in March - squeal! It will be the first end of treatment treat and the first visit abroad for us as a family in over four years. Shhhhhhhh, don't tell the children: http://www.christianlewistrust.org/

Saturday, 10th October 2015

Exhale. Operation Berthoud flu jab has been completed. Thanks to a fellow cancer mum for recommending a local pharmacy who offer a free walk-in flu jab service for those eligible. Also thanks to Andrew for having enough neutrophils, (unlike the last two weeks), in the window before steroids begin on Tuesday. Now to stop my paranoia that Andrew will accidentally have a nasal one at school with the rest of Year Two.

Tuesday, 13th October 2015

That time of the month again: vincristine chemo and steroids. Andrew and I are playing Monopoly waiting for our turn in the treatment room. Some poor mite is screaming, having a new NG tube fitted. After this month, we have only FOUR more pulses of vincristine and dexamethasone to go

Saturday, 17th October 2015

The last dexamethasone of October has gone down the hatch. Four months left. Five days a month to be done. Six tablets a day. One hundred and twenty tablets to go.

Friday, 23rd October 2015

I have another gorgeous bunch of flowers to adorn my kitchen table over half-term as a thank you for another conference. I had the most incredible day, seeing weeks of hard work come to life. It was inspiring to finish the day with the author, Anne Fine, talking about love of reading. I chatted with her whilst taking her to the station, all whilst wearing one blue shoe and one black shoe – whoops.

Friday, 30th October 2015

Thanks everyone for my birthday wishes. I had a day of two halves.

I got a parking ticket, but it was for £0.

We had lunch at Jamie's, but they forgot to cook my and Joseph's lunch so we got them for free.

I got lots and lots of lovely presents.

We saw 'Spectre' at the cinema.

We came home and Andrew had been sick everywhere. Poor pop.

Sunday, 1st November 2015

Thank you to everyone who ordered an Usborne Book or two (or ten). I have processed the order this morning and your books should be here by the end of the week. The final order was for £760.08 of books which means £456.05 of free books for the children at the Royal Marsden this Christmas. AWESOME! I will let you know what £1216.13 worth of books look like when they arrive!

Wednesday, 4th November 2015

One of my favourite days of the year! Usborne book order delivery day! The children have spent a merry hour sorting out the orders. All the books I chose are designed to cheer up, distract or entertain families during the long days in hospital, especially over Christmas.

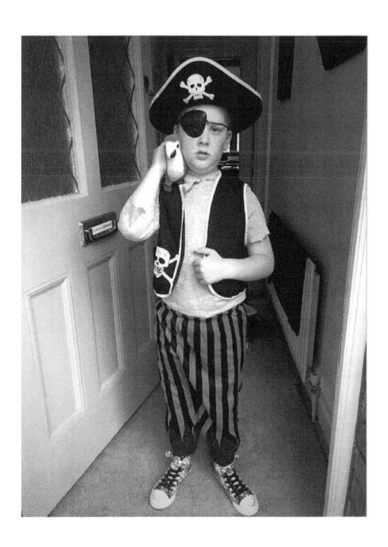

Chapter 18

Long Term Maintenance – Cycle 11

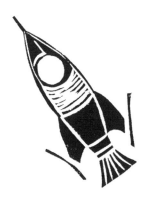

Cancer defined me

For three years or more now so

Who will I be next?

Tuesday, 10ᵗʰ November 2015
Another three months done. Andrew is still in remission and cancer-free.

We started Cycle Eleven today, which is three months long. We start Cycle Twelve, which is one month long, on 2ⁿᵈ February 2016.

Our official end of treatment date is Saturday 20ᵗʰ February 2016

Our last lumbar puncture is booked in for 16ᵗʰ February 2016.

We are allowing ourselves a little smile.

I dropped off this year's Usborne Books to the play team who were thrilled and very grateful. They took the '20 Christmas Cards to Colour' straight out of the box to give to a girl who has been told she has to be in isolation for six weeks. I have a very warm fuzzy feeling in my tummy.

Friday, 13ᵗʰ November 2015
It only cost £108 to upgrade our free travel insurance, which comes with our Nationwide bank account, to cover Andrew's medical conditions for a year and therefore our holidays in 2016. I am very pleased!

Tuesday, 24ᵗʰ November 2015 at 18:50
It is #CharityTuesday so I wanted to say:

Thank you to Cancer Research UK because without you my little boy would not be here today.

Thank you to Chartwell Cancer Trust as Clara has made friends for life with other siblings. I don't know what they talk about in our monthly meet ups but they share an unspoken bond that is the cancer experience.

Wednesday, 25th November 2015 at 14:10

I am excited. I have received a phone call from Starlight Children's Foundation. Would Andrew, plus one, like to come to our Christmas party at 11 Downing Street? YES, PLEASE!

Andrew's neutrophils are 0.2! That's low and means he has no immune system to fight off any illnesses going around. Boooooo. I don't want to end up in hospital. Bugs and germs, go away from us please and let Andrew stay well.

Friday, 27th November 2015

Never has a lumbar puncture at the Royal Marsden been so much fun, Michelle and Harrison. I am looking forward to Andrew's last one with you too. One thousand one hundred and fifty days done. Eighty-four to go. That is only 7% of the total left; we are 93% of the way there. I know of three people looking forward to finishing before us, nearing that 100%.

To those special people at the beginning of your cancer journey: you can do it. You will do it. You are strong enough. You will have awful days, but they will remind you to live and love the great days. You will make new friends for life. You will grow as a person and not quite be the same again, but you will be better for it. One day you will be 93% of the way there, thinking, how did that happen?

Sunday, 29th November 2015

The Bromley Child Cancer Support Group monthly meet ups finished 2015 on a high, with sixty members meeting today for the Churchill Theatre's pantomime. (Oh no you didn't!) A huge thank you to the Chartwell Cancer Trust for paying for our tickets, interval ice cream and a gift for each child. (They're behind you!) We laughed and laughed; it was a brilliant afternoon. (Oh, yes it was!) Utterly wonderful to see so much happiness on the faces of children (and parents) undergoing treatment. Hopefully everyone was able to suspend life for two hours and laugh. Always a pleasure to see everyone.

When I planned meet ups for 2015, I decided I didn't need a regular venue. I thought I would plan more party-style meets ups. After all, the 2014 pantomime had been such a huge success. I wanted each meet up to be a special time, full of great memories to help families get through the next month of treatment and procedures.

When I rang companies to book events and mentioned the support group and the reason for the group, people were more than generous. In January 2015 we had a private hire film screening at the Beckenham Odeon and all the adults had a free ticket. In March 2015 we had an Easter party at a hall in Knockholt with Mr. Marvel. The hall hire was reduced and the Mr. Marvel head office's commission was waivered. I booked a Pizza Express party in Beckenham for April and they offered to do it at zero cost. It is very hard to spend money once you mention children and cancer in the same sentence.

Tuesday, 1ˢᵗ December 2015 at 07:26

Team Berthoud are rather excited this morning, opening their advent calendars. This is our first winter since 2011 with no lengthy inpatient stays! Fingers crossed for the next month too.

Saturday, 5ᵗʰ December 2015

Twice a day, at the weekends, Andrew takes an antibiotic-type medicine to prevent pneumonia. Aged three, he took an instant dislike to the taste of the liquid, so we switched to tablet form. He had this crushed in anything we could hide it in and then eventually he swallowed the tablets cut up. For the last year or so he's had three quarters of a tablet, so a half and a quarter, but last month the dose was increased to a full tablet. Now Andrew swallows one Septrin tablet, slightly smaller than a five pence piece, whole, twice a day – he is remarkable!

Sunday, 6ᵗʰ December 2015

We had a wonderful day at Winter Wonderland, thanks to the Emily Ash Trust. The silent Disco was a big hit! I loved spending time with my cancer family, but left with feeling tinged by sadness that the end of our treatment may mean we see less of each other.

Tuesday, 8ᵗʰ December 2015

It is steroid week in the Berthoud household. Andrew and Daddy visited the local yesterday. Andrew has grown half a centimetre this month and lost a little weight too. Today was the last IV chemotherapy and steroids of 2015. Only two more to go. One thousand one hundred and sixty-one days done; seventy-four to go. That is only ten weeks!

Saturday, 12th December 2015

Joseph's homemade wreath is on the front door, the Christmas tree is up, the house is adorned and the children made mince pies, which are in the oven. I am feeling very thankful for all we have and I am very grateful to have all the Berthouds home and healthy.

Tuesday, 15th December 2015

This afternoon Andrew and I had the honour of going to 11 Downing Street for the Starlight Children's Foundation Christmas Party. The whole afternoon has been a once in a lifetime experience. We walked through the famous black gates and up to number 10 and then in through number 11. We were greeted by Danger Mouse, a princess and Karen Clifton! Upstairs there were crafts galore, and celebs galore: Janette Manrara, Joanne Clifton, Rupert Grint, John Newman, Lauren Murray, Brian Friedman, Nadiya Hussain, Geri Halliwell, Christian Horner, Lindsey and Radzi from Blue Peter, and of course, Father Christmas and George Osborne. Just as we were getting together for the big group photo, the Prime Minister appeared and Andrew leapt a mile! David disappeared off, but an aide ran after him to get his autograph for Andrew. I shook hands with everyone and thanked them for coming to make it so special for all of us. We got autographs (no photographs - we had to hand our phones in) of most people for Andrew and Clara. Everyone was totally down to earth and utterly charming. We have come away with two enormous bags of goodies, on top of the balloon hat and presents from Father Christmas, including a Red Bull cap, signed by Christian, eleven DVDs and a transformer. Spoilt rotten!

Friday, 18th December 2015

I am at home with my beautiful Mini Berthouds. I am so lucky to have two weeks with them now. Tonight we shall be celebrating getting through the whole of the autumn term with no unscheduled visits to hospital! Sixty-four days of chemo to go.

Sunday, 20th December 2015

Me and my big mouth. We are at the Queen Elizabeth Hospital, getting Andrew checked over after a temperature of 38.5 at home. Bloods have been taken. I am hoping there are enough neutrophils to allow us to come home.

Rats. Neutrophils are 0.5, so we are starting forty-eight hours of IV antibiotics for a viral infection. A nose swab and portable chest X-ray have been done. CRP is low, at 10. His chest X-ray is clear.

Monday, 21st December 2015

Morning all. We slept well, between 10pm and 5am. Andrew's temperature was 39.8, at 5am, when the nurse did his observations. He had some paracetamol, which took a while to take effect. He felt sick, thirsty and needed a wee, all at the same time. Eventually he fell back to sleep, with the windows wide open, and his temperature was 37.7 an hour later. He has woken up again and is happily watching Episode I of 'Star Wars'.

A massive thank you to Justin Tuck, from Fatboys Charity, who came to Woolwich today to deliver Andrew's gift to him. I am very grateful to Justin for taking time out of his own Christmas holiday to do a two-hour round trip to see us, and for changing venue at late notice due to our admission to hospital last night. Thank you, Fatboys, for your generosity. The Wii U is being set up as I type: http://www.fatboyscharity.co.uk/

At first we found asking for 'charity' uncomfortable. I found out about charities, big and small, through Facebook and the support groups. However, eventually I came to realise these charities were set up with the sole purpose of giving something back to families, like us, having a tough time. It makes the charities feel good to give, and it makes us feel grateful to receive. People are fundraising and working hard to raise money and, if we didn't ask for help, then their efforts would be unrewarded. I find a way of publically thanking the charities so they receive the publicity and awareness they deserve and can continue to help other families.

Andrew is still spiking temperatures of 39 or 40, so we will be here until Wednesday lunch time at least. His neutrophils have dropped to 0.3; his CRP is higher, up to 14. After another nap, we are now playing 'Mario Kart 8' on the Wii U again. I hear Father Christmas may pay us a visit soon! Nurse Chelsea is coming to the end of her twelve hour shift but staying to talk to the registrar who wants to add a third IV antibiotic to the mix. Andrew's had his maximum amount of paracetamol for the day, so if his temperature creeps up again, they'll give him IV fluids too. Stripped to his pants, windows open, fan on, and no sheet equals a grumpy Bear Berthoud, but hopefully we can get this under control.

Thanks to the support team at home for looking after Clara, allowing Joseph to go to Birmingham and sing with his choir. Night one and all. Have a BIG glass of mulled wine or red wine or mojito for me.

Tuesday, 22nd December 2015

Morning all. The junior doctor has been in. Neutrophils are stable at 0.3. Andrew's left ear is still looking very sore and inflamed, so it is very likely the cause of the high temperatures which continue. The rules have changed on Calpol doses at this hospital. They will now be permitted according to age, not weight. This means he has been having only half of what he could have had, according to his weight, so they're going to break the rules to give us a higher dose to try and knock the temperature on its head. His last temperature was 39.2 at 10am this morning, so we will stay for another forty-eight hours. It is getting rather close to Christmas! Andrew's wiped out after having three different antibiotics and being on an IV drip all night. I gave up on trying to go back to sleep after I was disturbed by the nurses for a fourth time, (quite rightly doing a brilliant job of looking after Andrew).

It is Joseph's turn to be in hospital for a day or so, so I am at home with Clara. I missed her. It has been a long forty-eight hours. It was lovely to see familiar faces for a grown up chat at the Queen Elizabeth today. Thanks too to the very wonderful Cath for the Perrott day of fun for Clara. Andrew's temperature was 38.1 as I left. Let that be the last now, please. Thank you to my parents who have rearranged Christmas to be in Beckenham instead of Suffolk - how wonderful!

When everything is in balance, life works. When one aspect goes wrong, like Andrew going into hospital, or Clara getting ill, or work getting busy, the scales unbalance. Joseph and I have had more than one conversation at three o'clock in the morning about who should take Andrew in to the hospital, based on whose meetings were the most important the next day.

I often go to work from the hospital, having to get dressed and smartened up in the shower room, after only a few hours disturbed sleep. Even if I am at home when Andrew is in hospital, I still have to get up for work, which means Clara has to go to someone's house for breakfast. When Andrew was an inpatient, during the conference, my mum came and slept in our house so Clara could stay in her bed and not be shipped off early. We inconvenience ourselves to benefit the children.

On these occasions the stress builds up and we get through the rough patches as best as we can, with the help of family, friends and neighbours. Andrew was only an inpatient, and really poorly, a few times. Most of the time he has viruses, which, if not for the cancer treatment, would not mean going to a hospital. Those times were the most frustrating. He would have high temperatures for days in a row due to a virus. Normally you would snuggle a child up on the sofa and dose them up with Calpol and Nurofen. For us though we have the separation and boredom of being in hospital.

Once the immediate stress is relieved, it lingers for a few days, or sometimes weeks, whilst we mentally catch up with ourselves, as well as the other parts of our life which have been neglected. Joseph spends a lot of time sacrificing sleep, whereas I am no use to anyone if I don't get at least seven hours.

I find comfort in routine, mundane tasks: putting a wash on, filling the dishwasher, walking around the supermarket or sitting with a coffee. I can spend time thinking about what is coming up and prioritising what needs to be done.

Wednesday, 23rd December 2015

Another 39.9 overnight. Seeing as all I want for Christmas is my boy to be home, I have donated £22.29 to Crisis UK, to enable someone without a home over Christmas, to have a day at a Crisis Shelter and a hot meal. This is a very annoying blip in the road, but we are still very lucky in many ways.

Thursday, 24th December 2015

Neutrophils are up a bit to 0.5. CRP 36. All other bloods looking good and his cultures are still negative. Andrew's temperature has been staying low since about 8pm yesterday. The large viral rash has now gone. Antibiotics are normally administered for five days so we'll still be in tomorrow. Thanks for all the afternoon Christmas joy, goodies and visits in the hospital. I am touched you took time out of your Christmas Eve to come and see us.

Okay, I am heartbroken now. Leaving the boys in the hospital was HARD. A part of me didn't believe that I would actually have to leave Andrew there on the most magical night of the year. I don't want to miss the moment Andrew sees he has a stocking at the end of his bed. (Andrew is still temperature free). We decorated Andrew's room with tinsel, fairy lights and mistletoe. He has hung his stocking up and put out a glass of sherry, a mince pie and a carrot.

I will snap out of it. A glass or two of my favourite Vouvray and some Twiglets will help. Enjoy your precious family time and special times. Merry Christmas from the Berthouds!

Friday, 25th December 2015
We are Home! Not out for a few hours but discharged and home for Christmas lunch.

Sunday, 27th December 2015
It has been forty-eight hours since we were discharged from the Queen Elizabeth, three naps and two good nights sleeps later, I feel like we can function and begin to enjoy what is left of the Christmas holidays. That was the most intensely stressful and difficult week of the year. On Christmas day, Clara woke at 6:30am, so we jumped into the car and drove straight to the Queen Elizabeth. She held onto her stocking for a whole hour before actually opening it with Andrew - she is AWESOME. She had made a pact with Andrew that they would only take two things out before being together. Gosh, I love them.

All of the staff were full of festive cheer: the play team, the cleaner, the cook, the nurses and the doctors. Father Christmas brought the children fake poo and a fake pencil in their stockings, much hilarity was had asking the nurses to clear up poo and write notes. Then the nurse tricked the doctor with the wobbly pencil too - I didn't dare! The registrar came to us first, at 9am, to say as we had been temperature-free for over forty hours; we could go home after the midday antibiotics - the best Christmas present ever. Unfortunately, the two other cancer patients on the ward were not allowed home, so we were (hopefully) discreet in our whooping. The CEO of the Trust came around mid-morning with (yet another) Father Christmas who was giving out gorgeous hand puppets. There was a lovely moment when the other boy on the ward bumped into Santa in the corridor and his face lit up on seeing HIM.

My Twitter feed went slightly bonkers with people wishing us well, and the DJ from Meridian radio, based in the Queen Elizabeth, offered Andrew a look around the studio, and even played a song for him on the radio. In short, it was horrid not all being together for the run up to Christmas, but the wonderful staff at the Queen Elizabeth Hospital made Christmas Eve and Christmas Day the best it could be and, to them, I would like to say thank you. If your child ever has to be in hospital over the festive period, rest assured, there will be a team of people in and out of the hospital, ready to make it special for you. Thank you to my social media network. You got us through a very tough week.

Wednesday, 30th December 2015

Andrew had a blood test this morning to see what's what after last week when everything crashed. He has had no daily chemotherapy for ten days and, of course, we are keen for him to have as much as possible as we approach the end of his treatment. His blood levels have bounced back nicely; those naughty neutrophils. which were 0.3 on Christmas Day, are now 2.1, and his platelets, which were low at 74, are now 215. Such a relief!

Wishing you all a happy and healthy 2016, with oodles of pleasant times and no nasty surprises. It will certainly be a whole new world for us.

Monday, 4th January 2016

We are at Queen Elizabeth Hospital. Back again. This is our last clinic at the Queen Elizabeth on treatment. Andrew is having his penultimate IV vincristine chemo and we start the penultimate steroids week. I'm so glad we've recovered from our week in hospital enough to cope with the emotions and lack of sleep steroids bring. Forty-seven days to go.

I had a moment on leaving: "Bye, Nurse Cat. See you? Oh my goodness, WE HAVE NO MORE APPOINTMENTS HERE." Andrew's last vincristine and dexamethasone is at the Royal Marsden. I lingered for a moment with images of previous visits and inpatient stays flashing through my head, then Andrew and I tried not to run out of the door to never come back.

Thursday, 7th January 2016

A little taste of the last twenty-four hours on steroids: yesterday Andrew got upset at having to go to school because he wanted to stay at home and be with his family (none of us were going to be at home). Having had pizza for dinner last night, he told me he was still hungry, on loop, for about an hour until he fell asleep. He slept for twelve hours last night but still woke up tired. Joseph had to carry him to school this morning, as he was upset: "I have no friends and no one plays with me!" This is not true. He stayed at school for half an hour, went to a podiatry appointment, then came home to sleep for an hour and a half. He has eaten his lunch and gone back to school again. Three more doses to go this week. Forty-four days of chemotherapy left.

Friday, 8th January 2016

12.30pm and we have only just managed to get Andrew to school. He burst in to tears at 8:55am and had to be brought home. He climbed back into bed and slept for two and a half hours. He woke up and ate his lunch, then Joseph carried him to school. He is still not very sure, but we got him in the building and scarpered out for lunch with a glass of wine.

Friday, 15th January 2016

In the beginning, after diagnosis, Andrew was poorly in isolation at the Royal Marsden. One day I walked past the four bed ward on my way to the parents' kitchen and noticed another mum with a similarly aged child. Said child also had hair, so I assumed he was at the beginning of his journey too. I remember asking the mum if she would like a cup of tea and some toast. All cancer parents will be able to tell you about the mums or dads and children they meet 'in the beginning' who become lifelong friends. Mine was Emma who, luckily, said yes to the tea and toast.

Today is 'the day' for Ollie: his last day of chemotherapy and 'the end'. I am so thrilled for you, so happy for you and so emotional, as it will be us soon and it feels scary!

Congratulations, Emma, Matthew, Daniel, Ollie and Stanley.

Saturday, 16th January 2016

I have started the process of turning the last three and a bit years into a book for Andrew and maybe, hopefully, it will be published. I haven't needed counselling, or medical support for depression. Writing the journey on Facebook is my counselling; it was my voice on the dark nights. Going to work was my break from the stress and, even though friends and family were amazed I continued to work, I needed to. It kept me sane.

The downside to Facebook is, when I am in the real world, I think most people know exactly what is going on in my life. Sometimes I feel under pressure to be as eloquent in real life as I am in type, but I'm not. I am tired, bumbling and emotional, barely holding it together for Andrew and Clara. As the years tick by, I forget some people are not on Facebook and so know nothing about what is going on.

Most importantly I want Andrew's story to help other families in the same situation as us. We had nothing to inform us at diagnosis of what it was really going to be like.

Tuesday, 19th January 2016

Oh dear. Andrew's blood results have dropped this week: neutrophils, 0.4, and platelets, low at 86. As the nurse said on the phone, the last time Andrew was off chemotherapy with low blood work, we were admitted for a week at Christmas. So no chemotherapy for a week and everything crossed he stays well. Please, please, PLEASE!

Thirty-two days to go.

Wednesday, 20ᵗʰ January 2016

Thirty-nine months completed. One month to go until End of Treatment on 20ᵗʰ February 2016. Is this real?

How wonderful on today of all days! Today both children received a Blue Peter badge in the post. When we met Lindsey and Radzi, from Blue Peter, at 11 Downing Street, in December, they suggested Andrew write in to explain how they had met each other, as he might be awarded a Blue Peter badge. He did so, as soon as we got home, but what the children didn't know is that I slipped in a letter with his picture.

Clara's letter from the editor says, "We recently received a lovely letter from your mummy, Melody. She told us how brilliant you have been whilst your brother, Andrew, has been receiving his treatment. The 'Blue Peter' team agree with your mum that you are an 'amazing sister who is kind and tender,' so we are awarding you a Blue Peter Badge".

Andrew's letter says, "We recently received a lovely letter from your mummy, Melody. She told us all about your bravery during your chemotherapy treatment and we're pleased to read that you are finishing treatment next month. The 'Blue Peter' team agree with your mummy that you are an 'amazing, brave, resilient, cancer-fighting champion,' so we are awarding you a Blue Peter Badge".

The children are thrilled. Joseph and I are very emotional partly with pride but also because we both wanted Blue Peter badges as children.

Monday, 25th January 2016

I have been asked a few times recently about how Andrew is feeling about the end of treatment. So I asked him at dinner. The truth is, he was diagnosed at three years and five months and the end of his treatment will be three years and four months later: half his life on treatment. He has no memories of life without cancer, hospitals and medicine. To put it into context:

I am thirty-nine, so it would be the same as my having had cancer treatment for the last nineteen and a half years. Or to put it another way, think about what you were doing during the London Olympics in 2012 as that is when we were blissfully cancer free.

So, to answer the question, he talked about what he is going to be losing: not seeing the nurses, not collecting beads of courage, not being able to park near to locations using the blue badge, and not visiting the hospital to play with the toys.

The two aspects he is excited about are: going on a plane and being able to run faster!

Tuesday, 26th January 2016

Andrew's neutrophils have risen to 0.7, but need to be 0.8 for him to restart chemotherapy, so we have another week off. I hope we get to start chemotherapy again so we can enjoy giving him the last one and stopping! Twenty-five days to go.

Friday, 29th January 2016

8am at the Queen Elizabeth Hospital.

We arrived at 4am after Andrew spiked a temperature, at home, of 39.1 at 3am. Completely out of the blue. He was fine yesterday! He woke us up at midnight, saying he had a very sore throat but was also very distressed and had a strange breathing pattern; he was struggling to catch his breath. It sounded like the stridor in a croupy cough but without the barking. We got him back to sleep, but then he woke up an hour later, very hot. He is still hot and shivery but also covered in a rash, with a few odd bruises on his hip and thigh, which might mean he has low platelets. A lovely Doctor was bleeped, from A&E, to come and look Andrew over. We finally fell asleep at 5.30am. IV antibiotics have been started.

Saturday, January 30th 2016

I am at home on Clara duty whilst the boys are in hospital. I had a lovely chat with the boys. Andrew is still temperature-free and coughing; he coughs when he is neutropenic. When I was in hospital, yesterday morning, speaking to Clara on the phone, she asked me if it was her fault Andrew was ill. Of course not, I said, and reassured her she had done NOTHING wrong. Interesting that she feels both guilt and responsibility. I am on antibiotics for a chest infection so it is possibly my fault or the fact there seem to be germs everywhere!

Andrew told me about an awesome dream he had where he had a mark on his forehead which meant he was a legendary flame bird who was great at gymnastics. Love them.

Andrew is looking a lot better this afternoon. He is off the fluid drip, which was used to bring his high heart rate down. He is therefore able to leave the room to play. We won't be discharged in time for the BCCSG January meet up in the morning, but he should be allowed out on day release to come along. The nurse is hopefully going to administer his IV antibiotics at 7am and 1pm, rather than 6am and 12pm. He has no neutrophils, at 0.0, so probably won't go to school on Monday.

Twenty-one days to go.

Sunday, 31st January 2016

I had a fabulous morning hosting January's BCCSG meet up at Build-a-Bear in Bromley.

It was "one of the best ever" meet ups, as all the children have been looking forward to it for weeks, with much excitement, and then all left clutching their teddy. We had two new families join us today, as well as the normal mixture of families, on and off treatment, so we have a real breadth of support.

Sibling to sibling.
Parent to parent.
Oncology child to child.

I think my favourite moment was when I caught an oncology child smiling for the first time in one of the meet ups.

Andrew was allowed out this morning for the meet up and I brought him back to the hospital for lunchtime IV antibiotics and to wait for the results of his blood cultures, which were due back at 8am. At 4pm, after sixty hours, (longer than the normal forty-eight) we found out the results were negative e.g. nothing had grown, which confirms Andrew has a virus (he's got a red throat, red ear and is snotty). We're switching to oral antibiotics, but because he still has 0.0 neutrophils, the Royal Marsden have said we have to stay in overnight, to check a switch to oral antibiotics doesn't make him spike a temperature. They will check his temperature every hour or so through the night. I am totally unprepared and have no overnight things or a phone charger (gasp!), as I thought I was bringing him home.

Twenty days to go.

Monday, 1st February 2016
Pinch punch first of the 'end of treatment' month and no returns.

We slept well. No temperatures caused by the antibiotic. However, he is itchy and the antibiotics could be causing the rash on his head and neck, so we have been discharged and are at home with no antibiotics. The oncology consultant looked Andrew over this morning and decided, in light of his viral symptoms and the reaction to the antibiotics, that no more antibiotics were needed. She apologised for us having to stay in for another night and said she would have allowed us home yesterday if asked. Never mind.

At home mean Mummy gave Andrew some maths to do, whilst I sat and did some work. A maths investigation with Smarties wasn't fun enough though - so he stomped off crying and is now fast asleep on the sofa. Pooped Pop. Nineteen days to go

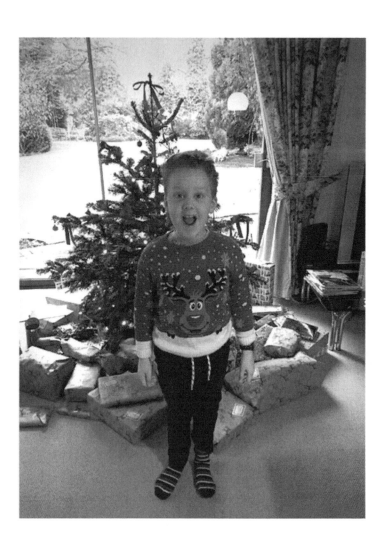

Chapter 19

Long Term Maintenance – Cycle 12

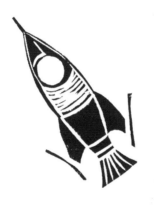

Leukaemia's gone

In remission finally

Our life is reborn

Tuesday, February 2nd 2016

Another twelve weeks done and still in remission. We were at the Royal Marsden this morning to start Cycle Twelve and to meet Andrew's consultant.

Andrew also had his last IV vincristine chemo through his Wiggly.

We have picked up his last bag of drugs from pharmacy.

Andrew has started his last steroid week. A momentous day!

One thousand two hundred and seventeen days since diagnosis.

Eighteen days to go.

Wednesday, 3rd February 2016

Last Wednesday on steroids.

Last Day Two of steroids.

Last trip to Pizza Express on steroids (Two for One Wednesdays)

Will Andrew ever eat one of their pizzas again?

Seventeen days to go.

Thursday, February 4th 2016

It is 'World Cancer Day', but it is also 'Germ Catcher Super Hero Day' in Year Two at Andrew's school.

Andrew's neutrophils were 0.2 at the Royal Marsden on Tuesday, so we're guessing, with steroids, they have risen enough now for him to go in.

He wanted to be 'The Leukaemia Catcher', so is dressed as a doctor, with a pen in his top pocket, a watch on his wrist, a stethoscope around his neck and a medical bag full of blood bottles, hand sanitiser, rubber gloves and, most importantly, stickers for good patients.

LAST Day Three on steroids

LAST Thursday on steroids

Sixteen days to go.

Friday, 5th February 2016

Well we did it. Today is the last school day Andrew will have to do on steroids. He woke up (in my bed, after arriving in the middle of the night, depressed and lonely) and started saying, "I don't want to go to school. I'm going to be tired."

It was a two-man mission to get him dressed, out the door and in the line, and there was a moment when I thought it would all go horribly wrong, but he queued up behind a friend and happily followed his classmates in.

LAST Friday on steroids

LAST Day Four on steroids

Fifteen days to go.

I have had an incredible day off with big plans! I met the oncology nurse at Croydon University Hospital (CUH) this morning, along with Michael Douglas from the Chartwell Cancer Trust. The nurse is new and keen to set up a support group for Croydon families. A Croydon Mum told her about the BCCSG so she emailed Michael who has agreed to fund a support group in Croydon too.

We had a tour of the paediatric ward in CUH, and golly, we are so lucky at the Queen Elizabeth in Woolwich. Croydon only have one oncology room, no kitchen for parents and no separate playroom for oncology children. Three years ago I didn't think I would be saying the facilities at Queen Elizabeth are amazing - but wow they are!

I have agreed to set up a Croydon Childhood Cancer Support Group (CCCSG) and get it going using my Bromley model. I decided to have separate meet ups in Croydon, rather than inviting the families to join in with BCCSG. I think this will be easier, especially for families who do not drive. We are starting with a Build-a-Bear meet up in March, which was a big hit with the Bromley children.

The downside to running support groups is constantly hearing of children who are diagnosed and suffering with a cancer diagnosis. Every new diagnosis or relapse stabs me in the heart; it catapults me back to our own diagnosis day. It is tremendously hard, constantly hearing about children with cancer, but what keeps me motivated is the difference the Chartwell Cancer Trust and the support groups make to these families. The smiles on the children's faces say it all and stay with me, as does knowing that, for another month, they will have something happy to remember whilst undergoing treatments.

The meet ups are more than just a few hours, once a month, talking. They are the creation of a whole support network across Bromley, of people being on the end of the phone or on the Internet when needed. They are counselling for all of us.

For me, they are knowing that someone understands how I feel, even without having to say so. They are not being afraid to ask the daft questions. We can all learn from each other and get hope and strength for the long dark days, because someone else already has.

It feels fantastic that something good has come out of Andrew's diagnosis of leukaemia. I am able to give something back.

P.S. Andrew is fast asleep in bed at home - he lasted until 1.30pm.

Saturday, 6th February 2016
Andrew is back in bed and fast asleep, after waking up at 6am. Hopefully he will have a long sleep now, ready for an energetic trampolining party this afternoon.

Today should have been the last day of steroids, but it seems we forgot to give him his afternoon dose on Wednesday - how stupid! No wonder he was okay about going into school on Thursday morning! So now we have to give him this last extra dose on Sunday morning.

Last Saturday on steroids.

At dinner Clara asked us how we knew Andrew had cancer. We explained about the symptoms and the lead up to diagnosis.

She then asked how we knew which type of cancer it was. Andrew chipped in with a comment, which I asked him to repeat. He said, "Whether it was a killing cancer or leukaemia". My heart broke in two. I explained about the Bone Marrow Aspirate procedure, which occurred 'in the beginning', which told us if it was ALL, AML, CLL or CML.

Naive of me, I suppose, to think he didn't know people died of cancer. I realised I had made a mistake, when talking to him about David Bowie dying, and he asked me what of. I told him 'cancer', but that it was a different type to his.

Clara then asked me whether she had changed since Andrew was first poorly. I thought she meant in the same way that Andrew's hair had changed from blonde and curly to dark and straight. She meant "As a person, have I changed?'

I told her we had all changed during this experience, and she is so kind, caring and resilient, and she will be an extraordinary grown up because of these experiences.

She said she thought the experience had made her more independent.

I told her she looks for the good in each situation and is wonderful when plans have to change at the last minute. She agreed and said, "Like Christmas. That was upsetting."

She said she wouldn't have met fellow cancer siblings, Lily or Eden, if it weren't for the cancer, and she is glad that she did. I have wondered whether there will be a point when Clara will suddenly realise how much we have been through as a family, and what Andrew being diagnosed with cancer meant. I suppose this is the beginning of a lot of questions both of them will ask Joseph and me.

Fourteen days to go.

Sunday, 7th February 2016

We made it! Last steroid! The Steroid Rocket is full. Blast off! Bye dexamethasone, we will not miss you one jot. What a relief! There will be no bottle-smashing party, as our dex comes in a blister pack, so instead, we threw the packets away with a flourish.

Thirteen days to go.

Monday, 8th February 2016

Andrew was a sad bunny this morning. The steroids mean he has been sleeping badly, having nightmares and ending up in bed with me. One vivid dream was about being on a plane: all his favourite teddies flew out of the window and got chopped up in the propellers.

He is tired from the steroids, tired from the nightmares and tired from the insomnia. He was particularly upset this morning, as Daddy was in Southampton, enjoying the Super Bowl, and Clara hadn't done her homework, so I was giving her all my remaining attention whilst making breakfast, making packed lunches and emptying the dishwasher.

Then the 'fear' of school kicked in. It has lingered on from his depression, whilst on steroids, last week. I got him to school; he snivelled into my coat whilst waiting for the bell to go. All would be well, I thought to myself, when his teacher came out. The bell rang and then a supply teacher walked towards the line - oh no! Luckily the class 1:1 was there and I asked for help. She was brilliant and took Andrew away, saying they were "going to do something fun - come and help me."

I turned around and walked away, trying not to burst into tears, and repeating in my head, "We won't have to do this again." If and when I am back, working in schools, I shall try and remember this moment and how I, as the parent, would love to have been sent an email or text to say he had settled and was happy.

Twelve days to go.

Wednesday, 10th February 2016
Are you ready to count with me? TEN!
Last oral methotrexate.

Every Wednesday evening, Andrew has a chemotherapy drug called methotrexate – the amount of tablets he takes has increased over the years, but tonight he will be taking nine. Next Wednesday, he won't be having any, as he will have the same drug injected directly into his spinal fluid during a lumbar puncture on Tuesday.

Ten days to go.

Thursday, 11th February 2016
NINE! Nine days to go.

When Andrew finishes this journey he will have had:
1235 days of treatment
Around 1150 days of chemotherapy
25 General Anaesthetics,
23 Lumbar Punctures
22 bags of blood or platelets.
73 nights in hospital, 62 of which were at the Queen Elizabeth
And around 60 days of missed schooling.
We have also directly raised £9000 for various cancer charities

Friday, 12th February 2016
EIGHT! Last day at school for Andrew whilst 'on treatment'.

Eight days to go.

Saturday, 13th February 2016
SEVEN! One week to go. Seven days to go.

In three months' time Andrew's portacath will be removed. This was inserted on the 9th October 2012 and unusually Andrew still has the original portacath inside him. They made an incision in his side and his neck to implant it. They will go in through the same scar on his neck to remove it.

This portacath has always been very mobile (moves around when nurses want to hold onto it) and is now much deeper inside him than at first as he has grown from a 3 year old to a 7 year old around it.

When they implanted the portacath they cut the nerve endings directly under the skin to minimise pain on accessing. Andrew also has numbing cream or cold spray to help with the pain of a needle being pushed through his skin.

The nurses accessed his port weekly for bloods, every time he was admitted to hospital with a temperature to administer antibiotics and for IV chemo. The area of skin above the port is now scarred from the hundreds and hundreds of needles having been pushed through it.

Andrew used to have to be held still on my lap to be accessed whilst screaming, arms flailing. I would hold his arm up and over his head, with him telling me not to hold his hand and me saying "I'm not" whilst I was actually holding my fingers in a thumb and forefinger pincer around his wrist ready to grab if he moved.

One afternoon early on in his treatment he head butted me and bruised (probably broke) my nose as he flung his head backwards during an accessing. My eyes streamed and I cried quietly, due to the pain, whilst the nurse accessed him; she could see me but he was facing away. I pulled myself together enough that when it was over he couldn't see me with tears rolling down my cheeks.

Over time he became used to being accessed and would sit nicely on my lap enjoying the cuddle and eventually he didn't need me at all. He did however need to be in control of the needle all the way through treatment and would count down from 5 to 1 to prepare himself.

When the port wouldn't give out blood we had various tricks to try:
Arm up over head
Stand up
Flap arms like a chicken
Big fake cough

However sometimes we just had to take out the 'Mr Wonky' and reaccess with a new Mr Wiggly, a much better option than digging the needle around inside him trying to get it into the right place in the port. Doing that would make him scream and cry.

So bye bye Bubble – thank you for being a part of Andrew for 3 years and 8 months and for being a vital piece of life saving tech.

Sunday, 14ᵗʰ February 2016
SIX!

We had lunch with NCT friends in Wivenhoe and then drove down to the 02 for the 'Strictly Come Dancing' Live show!

'Strictly Come Dancing' has been such a big part of our cancer journey, especially for Clara. More so for Andrew after meeting Karen, Jeanette and Joanne at 11 Downing

Street before Christmas. I must admit, when Georgia and Gio came on to do the first dance, I gave a little happy cry and then Jay did that JIVE!

Last Sunday on chemotherapy. Six days to go.

Monday, 15th February 2016

Big breath. Ready? FIVE! One thousand two hundred and thirty days since diagnosis.

Five days to go.

Last Monday on chemotherapy.

Last community nurse visit on treatment (they'll still come for a while after).

Tuesday, 16th February 2016

FOUR!

Last lumbar puncture to check for cancerous cells in his spinal fluid (the twenty-third time he has had this procedure)

Last nil-by-mouth and general anaesthetic on treatment (one more needed for his portacath to be removed in a few months' time)

Last time I have to sign the form acknowledging all the horrid potential side effects, unable to say 'no'

Last chemotherapy injection into his spinal fluid

Last visit to the Royal Marsden on treatment

Last Wiggly access on treatment (hopefully)

Last beads of courage being collected from the play team

Last Tuesday on chemotherapy

I am a bit scared and nervous. Four days to go.

G'ah! Andrew woke up and ate a sneaky bag of haribo at 6.30am! The rule is that we have to wait for six hours after food before having a general anaesthetic.

Andrew is back (still waiting for food) with a souvenir mask from the anaesthetist. Andrew had no idea what the mask was, as he is asleep when they put it over his nose and mouth. He was wide-eyed when we told him!

Wednesday, 17th February 2016
THREE! Last Wednesday on chemotherapy. Three days to go.

Things I didn't know about cancer diagnosis:
1. I had heard of Leukaemia and when I told the GP Andrew's symptoms I suspected that they added up to Leukaemia - but I didn't know Leukaemia was cancer. I thought it was just another childhood illness that some kids got.
2. I didn't know you could get a cancer that you couldn't feel as a lump or see in a scan. I thought all cancers could be 'cut out' like breast cancer - so how do you cut out bad blood cells? You cannot of course which is why the treatment for Leukaemia is so long.
3. I didn't know chemo was just 'medicine' and could be taken in tablet form anywhere.
4. I didn't know it was possible to have chemo and not be sick or lose your hair. The intensive chemo made Andrew's hair fall out and throw up every day for 9 months. However, for two and a half

years after this the maintenance chemotherapy just kept things at bay whilst he looked every inch the 'normal' little boy with a mop of crazy hair.

5. I didn't know when your hair fell out, that it fell out everywhere. Andrew lost the hair on his head but also on his face his eyebrows, eye lashes and leg hair. I was so fixated on his bald head that I didn't notice the rest until they started to grow back.

6. I didn't know that cutting hair short makes it harder for you to pick out of food when the hair starts falling out.

7. I didn't know general anaesthetics could only last for 10 minutes. I also didn't know that grownups with Leukaemia have Lumbar Punctures without a general anaesthetic as they are only used to ensure the child doesn't move during the procedure.

8. I didn't know it was possible to go through such a traumatic experience as a family and come out stronger, more resilient and grateful for the things that the journey has taught us.

Thursday, 18th February 2016
TWO!

I have counted up all of Andrew's beads of courage since threading on the new ones, collected on Tuesday, and he has two thousand four hundred and sixty-six in total, but the all-important two thousand four hundred and sixty-seventh purple heart bead is waiting to be collected and threaded on after our first check up in April 2016. LAST Thursday on Treatment.

Two days to go.

Friday, 19th February 2016
ONE!

One day more until 20th February 2016.
One day more until a new 'normal' can begin.
One day more until I 'was' a cancer mummy.
One day more until my son 'had' cancer.

I love 'Les Miserables'. I took twelve friends to see the film on January 13th 2013, three months after Andrew's diagnosis, to say thank you for everything they had done for us. I knew nothing about the storyline.

I drove around for months afterwards listening to the soundtrack, and Cath even took me to see the play the following November, for my birthday.

(Adapted from Les Mis)
Another day
Another destiny
A Never Ending road to being Cancer Free
One day more to a new beginning,
There's a new world
For the winning
One more dawn,
One more day,
One day more!

LAST Friday on chemotherapy.
One day to go.

Saturday, 20th February 2016
ZERO!

Today is the day,
We have reached zero,
We have reached 100%,
We have reached our target,
We have crossed the finish line,
The rocket has landed safely,
We did it!

Cancer 0 Berthouds 1
Andrew is a cancer-fighting champion!
Thank you everyone for your never ending support on the journey.
Thank you for being there with us as we reach the end, cheering us on from the side lines.
Thank you to Cancer Research UK, for ensuring Andrew is alive today and with fewer long-lasting side effects.
Thank you, NHS, for three years of world class paediatric oncology service.
Thank you to all the doctors, nurses and anaesthetists for keeping my little boy alive during the days, nights and at weekends too.
Last Saturday on chemotherapy.

Last day of chemotherapy.

0 days to go.

We did it.

We beat leukaemia.

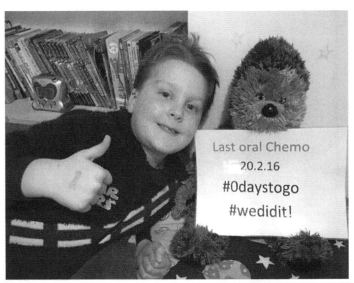

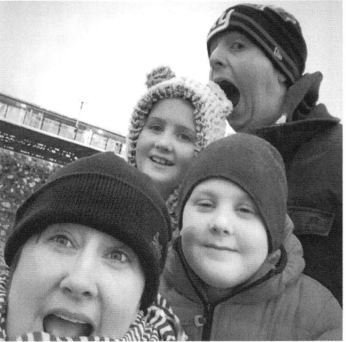

"When you ride a good rocket ship to orbit, you have a lot to be thankful for"

Bill Shepherd – NASA Astronaut

Acknowledgements

A huge thank you has to go to the following people who backed my Kick Starter project and are therefore responsible for making the book come alive. The successful funding of this project enabled me to edit and design We Beat Leukaemia.

Allison Longley
Sarah and Mike Bennett
Christine Stephen
Naomi Ward
Katie Jackson
Rhian Arrenberg
Hannah and Jean Paul Lebon
Sarah Bullock
Matthew & Holly Jackson
Larissa Apsley
The Glover Family
Michelle Phillips
Charlotte Searle
Laura James
Joanne Conduit-Smith
James Taylor-Nye
Judy Taylor
Helen Kirwan
Ruth Stebbings
Gaye Endler

Emma Harrison
Nina Morris
Kirstie Fulthorpe
Galya Holden
Andrea Hart
Chris Barrell
Debbie and Paul Court
Michelle Hakim
Amanda Schofield
Simon & Joy Lang
Amanda and Graeme Davies
Nadia O'Hare
Kirsten Abbott
Sam and Ross Sharland
Alison Taylor
Natalie Taylor
The Hall Family
Sarah Kazakos
Anna Young
Kerri Baker
Penny O'Sullivan
Denise Walker
Andy Szebeni
Cath and Dan Perrott
Michelle Njuguna-Arscott
Sian and Charles Maragna
Robin Bosher
Sanad Saif Abukishk
Shaun Jarrett Smith
Jo Townsend
Michelle Simpson
Chuon-Szen Ong
Sam Schofield

Bernadette Telford
Lucy Milmo
Andy and Polly Cross
Shelley Kavanagh
Rebecca Hurst
Elaine Alford
Jane McAlpine
Katie Kidd
Helen Maclean
Maria Scrivens
Alahree and Hopeton McDonell-Reid
Betty Johnson

My thanks also go to:

Lisa Roberts for telling me again and again that I should write a book.

Zelda Burbourgh for reading the first draft and seeing the potential within. Thank you for your words of wisdom and for helping me choose a title when I couldn't see the wood for the trees.

Nathalie Andrews for your Girl and Cat editing skills - ありがとう.

Helen Aida and Esther Pilger – your finding time in your busy lives to read and edit the manuscript made the book what it is today.

All the fellow cancer mummies including Beth Bumpking, Charlotte Charles and Kerry Brown who read my early drafts. Your interest in the book and feedback kept me motivated and was the drive I needed to keep writing.

Helen Maclean and Shaun Jarrett Smith, thank you for your invaluble support through the maze of crowdfunding.

Lisa Wooldridge, thank you for taking the time to create a beautiful piece of artwork for the cover of the book.

Lastly to Clara and Andrew – thank you for never giving up. You taught me to look for the best in everything and to enjoy every moment. I love you.

Websites

http://cclasp.co.uk
http://chartwellcancertrust.co.uk
http://chartwellcancertrust.co.uk/tiger-ward
http://coffee.macmillan.org.uk
http://uk.theodora.org/en-gb
http://www.bakingasmile.org
http://www.bechildcanceraware.org
http://www.childrenwithcancer.org.uk
http://www.christianlewistrust.org
http://www.clicsargent.org.uk
http://www.cyclistsfc.org.uk
http://www.emilyashtrust.co.uk
http://www.fatboyscharity.co.uk
http://www.forwardfacing.co.uk
http://www.lucysdaysout.org
http://www.macmillan.org.uk/information-and-support/leukaemia/acute-lymphoblastic-all
http://www.merlinmembership.co.uk/disabled.html
http://www.merlinsmagicwand.org
http://www.roundtable.co.uk
http://www.starlight.org.uk
http://www.yourheromadesuper.com
https://www.bloodwise.org.uk
https://www.ceacard.co.uk
https://www.royalmarsden.org

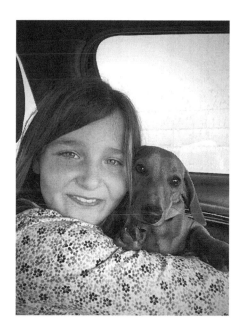

Front cover design by Lisa Wooldridge

Erin was diagnosed with Acute Lymphoblastic Leukaemia in May 2013. She finished treatment in August 2015. She is our hero and a very brave and strong young girl. I met Melody and Andrew at the Royal Marsden, Melody with her easy smile and comforting advice made us feel better immediately. Art has been my therapy whilst Erin has been having treatment so I jumped at the chance to be part of Melody's book and design a cover for her.

https://m.facebook.com/lisawoolart/
www.lisartist.com

Printed in Great Britain
by Amazon